S.K. Kulishov

OXYMORON LIKE PATHOLOGY: MECHANISMS, DIAGNOSIS, TREATMENT CORRECTION

2018

POLTAVA

OXYMORON LIKE PATHOLOGY: MECHANISMS, DIAGNOSIS, TREATMENT CORRECTION

Kulishov S.K.

POLTAVA 2018

Kulishov S.K. OXYMORON LIKE PATHOLOGY: MECHANISMS, DIAGNOSIS, TREATMENT CORRECTION. – 103 p.

The principles of oxymoron like pathology diagnosis and treatment correction were presented in this monograph. Some directions, algorithms were offered.

ISBN - 13: 978-1724677419

ISBN - 10: 1724677411

Introduction

It's known, that oxymorons are a proper subsets of the expressions, whose values mutually exclusive, and give us a semantic paradox [1,2].

We proposed and tested algorithms for diagnosis of oxymoron like pathology, as prerequisite for treatment correction [1,2].

Oxymoron like syndromes, diseases, multimorbidity, aging and aging dependent pathology are fragments of scientific investigations by some projects:

- «Oxymoron, fractal, anti-fractal, Moebius strip like pathology: mechanisms, diagnosis, treatment», ResearchGate [3,4,5,6,7], [https://www.researchgate.net/profile/Sergii_Kulishov2].

- «Psychological features, stress sensitivity, emotional intelligence of the patients with oxymoron, fractal, anti-fractal, Moebius strip like pathology as additional basis for diagnosis and treatment decision making», ResearchGate [7], [https://www.researchgate.net/profile/Sergii_Kulishov2].

- «Creative clinical thinking as derivative of multiplicity of intelligence forms: principles, training», ResearchGate [8], [https://www.researchgate.net/profile/Sergii_Kulishov2].

References

1.Kulishov S.K., Yakovenko O.M., Tretiak N.G. Training for creative thinking as a derivative of system and antisystem comparison, prerequisites for the mathematical modeling. Proceedings of the ICL conference 22.09.- 25.09.2009, the Kassel University Press; 2009, 71-73.

2. Kulishov S.K., Iakovenko O.M., Tretiak N.G. Clinical thinking training as a derivative of system and antisystem comparison, precondition to increase creativity of medical students, physicians. Proceedings of the ICL conference (Hasselt, Belgium) 15.09.-17.09.2010, the Kassel University Press, 2010, 337-343.

3. Bobrov V.A., Kulishov S.K. The adaptive ischemic and reperfusion syndromes in the patients with ischemic heart disease: mechanisms, diagnosis, substantiation of therapy. Poltava: Dyvosvit, 2004, 240 p.

4. Kulishov S.K., Iakovenko O.M. Solving clinical problems using system and anti-system comparison, graphic modeling. J. Innovative Medicine and Biology, 2011, 2-3: 30-42.

5. Kulishov S.K., Iakovenko O.M. Moebius strip like pathology: mechanisms, diagnosis, treatment correction. Proceedings of the 2015 international conference on health informatics and medical systems (HIMS 2015), ed. H.A. Arabnia, L. Deligiannidis, WORlDCOMP'15, Las Vegas, USA. (July 27-30, 2015), CSREA Press, 2015, 36-40.

6. Bobyryov V. M., Kulishov S.K., Vakhnenko A. V., Vlasova O.V. Genetic algorithm for making pharmacotherapy decision in the patients with multimorbidity. Wiad Lek, 2017; 71, 6 cz. I: 1142-1145.

7. Kulishov S.K., Iakovenko O.M., Shvedenko A.G., Shaposhnyk O.A., Kudria I.P., Bublyk O.O. Aging as result of racemic oxymoron, fractal and anti-fractal, Moebius strip like processes. Poltava, ResearchGate, 2018, 75 p.

8. Kulishov S.K., Iakovenko O.M. Training of creative clinical thinking as derivative of multiple intelligence manifestations. Poltava, ReseachGate, 2017. - 92 p.

Chapter 1. Principles of oxymoron like pathology diagnosis

1.1. Oxymoron pathology diagnosis as a derivative of system and antisystem comparison

Prerequisites of solving clinical problem using system and anti-system comparison [1,2]

Basis of our creative solving method is necessary to compare the elements systems and antisystems [1,2]. The algorithm consists from [1,2]:

- Formulation of the goal of creative task;

- Formulation thesis (or antithesis), which are key in solving the problem;

- Formulation of antithesis (or thesis), which blocks the solution to achieving the goal;

- Introduction thesis and antithesis as an adjective-noun combination of preliminary oxymorons-solutions. Oxymorons are a proper subset of the expressions called contradictions in terms. The most common form of oxymoron involves an adjective-noun combination.

Systemic solving is used to implement the goals of the creative task [1,2,3]. Analytical stage of systemic thinking [1,2,3] is aimed at listing as much, as possible components [1,2,3], constituent elements, sub-thesis and sub-antithesis [1,2,3]. Synthetic stage of systemic thinking [1,2,3] was characterized by grouping them into system-antisystem complexes, the compositions, finding a central, common theme through the understanding of sub-themes [1,2,3].

Grouping sub-themes is focusing efforts to overcome the cognitive dissonance, the formulation of intermediate and final decisions, the development of abilities, skills to recruit and use of system solutions [1,2,3]. System thinking can be used to achieve systemic focus in situations for which there are one or more sets of decisions [1,2,3]. The nature of the creative task causes the using of mathematical, physical, chemical, biological, visual tools [1,2,3].

Algorithmic thinking is represented in the human population is irregularly, which affects the quality of learning programming [1,2,3]. The ability to write algorithms to understand their nature and logic of the software is useful for various professionals, including the physicians [1,2,3].

The algorithm is a system of operations to convert data in the result as a generalized solution [1,2,3]. Solving unfamiliar tasks require the efforts of search algorithms [1,2,3]. The presence of efficient algorithms for solving problems which are before, contributes to a positive outcome [1,2,3]. Values of heuristics, algorithms for solving creative problems continue growing [1,2,3].

The aim of our work is solving clinical problems by system and anti-system comparison [1,2].

The methodology of clinical creative solving, as the derivative of the system and antisystem comparisons

Proposed and tested the algorithm for creative thinking as derivative of system and antisystem comparison for solving clinical problems of the multimorbidity, syndromes of the consumption [1,2,4]. Algorithm of creative thinking boils down to: formulation of the goal of creative tasks, the formation of the set thesis and the antithesis, thesis and antithesis versions of oxymorons, the transformation of intermediate oxymorons in the final creative decisions [1,2].

The methodology of the algorithm for creative thinking [1,2,3,4,5]:

A. Formulation of the goal of creative task -

- Formulation thesis and antithesis, which are key in solving the problem and its blocking;

- Formulation of thesis-antithesis preliminary oxymoron solution of creative task.

B. Analytic thinking -

- Formulation subthesis and subantithesis, which are keys in solving creative task and its blocking;

C. Synthetic thinking as search of central theme -

- Grouping constituent elements into system and antisystem complexes, the compositions;

- Formulation of oxymorons from system and antisystem complexes as subthemes;

- Unification of oxymorons as subthemes in the general oxymoron theme, solution through fractal structures, focusing- defocusing for overcoming of limiting.

Some illustrations of results achieved by using oxymoron like algorithm for creative solving clinical problems

Examples of the results of our algorithms for creative solving are [1,2,6]:

- Formulation of the goal of creative tasks: to determine the role of coronary and peripheral ischemia-reperfusion in the patients with ischemic heart disease;

- Formulation thesis: myocardial ischemia-reperfusion;

- Formulation antithesis: peripheral distance post-ischemic reperfusion;

- Introduction thesis-antithesis oxymorons-solutions: diagnosis of systemic effects of ischemia- reperfusion, the availability of stunned, hibernation myocardium due to the consumption of anti-ischemic, antireperfusion factors of protection from the negative influences in the patients with ischemic heart disease.

The protective precondition of the cardiovascular system to peripheral post-ischemic reperfusion in the patients with stable stable angina of effort is characterized by an adequate and redundant response of the systemic hemodynamics after decompression of extremities [1,2,6]. The protective precondition is more often observed in the patients with stable angina of effort of the I-II class than of the III, and reflects the optimal current of disease [1,2,6].

Criteria of diagnostics of lowering of anti-reperfusion protection of the heart in the patients with IHD were the expressed deterioration of the central hemodynamics to modeling of peripheral ischemia, reperfusion [1,2,6].

Formulation of sub-goal of creative tasks: to determine the role of peroxidation-antioxidant system in the pathogenesis of coronary heart disease [1,2,6]. Formulation: subthesis - lipid peroxidation; sub-antithesis - antioxidant protection [1,2,6]; Submission of solutions: diagnosis of syndromes by consumption of prooxidant and antioxidant factors due to myocardial ischemia-reperfusion in the patients with acute myocardial infarction [1,2,6].

A generalized algorithm for diagnosis of consumption syndromes is reduced to determining the ratio of pro-gradient and anti-gradient factors, i.e. those that contribute to or block the development of pathological process: raising pro-gradient and anti-gradient factors are characteristic of the initial stage, followed by an overwhelming increase in one of them, and then decline in the level of both as pro-gradient and anti-gradient factors [1,2,6]. We have determined that coagulopathy consumption syndrome (syndrome of disseminated intravascular coagulation - SDIC) is just one manifestation of interaction coagulation and anticoagulant system [1,2,6]. Similar nature is possible for reactions of peroxide and antioxidant systems as peroxidation consumption syndrome [1,2,6]. The basis of peroxidation consumption syndrome is lipolytic process [1,2,6]. Proteolytic pathogenesis is typical for the patients with syndrome of disseminated intravascular coagulation [1,2,6]. And if SDIC syndrome characterized by two opposing processes - increase blood clotting (thrombosis) and fibrinolytic activation (hemorrhage), the peroxidation consumption syndrome accompanied by similar changes of pro-oxidation (foci with high lipid peroxidation - LPO) and antioxidant response (foci with marked antioxidant effect) [1,2,6]. This syndrome characterized by the formation of a set of primary and secondary centers of consumption: one - antioxidants, others – prooxidants [1,2,6]. This result leads to activation and blocking of lipolysis, phospholipolisis, intravascular peroxidation cells (platelets, leukocytes) and plasma factors of blood (ceruloplasmin, iron, pyretic proteins) [1,2,6]. Consumption of basic substrate of LPO, antioxidants contribute complicated course of disease, concomitant deterioration of lipid-dependent diseases [1,2,6].

Thus, our algorithm of creative thinking is a technique for gaining systemic insights into complex problems [1]. It will help everyone create a mental framework for understanding the systemic and anti-systemic thinking concept [1,2,6].

Systemic effects post-ischemic reperfusion in the patients with coronary atherosclerosis, peripheral and carotid arteries may result from consumption syndromes [1,2,6]. Last reflect interaction between reperfusion and protect against negative effects of reperfusion, including peroxidation and antioxidant protection, pro-coagulation and fibrinolytic activity [1,2,6].

The use of systemic thinking has been used to achieve a systemic focus on multimorbidity (a combination in the patients with ischemic heart disease, essential hypertension, diabetes mellitus second type and pancreatobiliary pathology) as a reflection of aggregate consumption syndromes of pro-inflammation and anti-inflammation, antioxidant and pro-oxidation, pro-ischemic and anti-ischemic, reperfusion and anti-reperfusion factors [1,2,6].

A new direction in the cardiology is based on the concept the effects, syndromes of the consumption as a common biological principle of desadaptation and diagnosis of the viable, stunned, hibernation myocardium and cardiac protective precondition on the basis of biochemical, instrumental, mathematical modeling [1,2,6].

Algorithms of individual diagnostic and treatment solving were presented on the examples of patients with ischemic heart disease, ischemic-reperfusion syndrome [1,2,6], pro-arrhythmic effects of antiarrhythmic drugs, pro-ischemic effects of anti-ischemic drugs [1,2].

Oxymorons, as a combination of adjectives and nouns antonyms, are characteristics of symptoms, syndromes and diseases [1,2].

Conclusion

The algorithms, principles, steps of creative thinking, solving clinical problems by system and anti-system comparison are presented in this part of.

References

1. Kulishov S.K., Iakovenko O.M. Solving clinical problems using system and anti-system comparison, graphic modeling. J. Innovative Medicine and Biology, 2011, 2-3: 30-42.

2.Kulishov S.K., Iakovenko O.M., Shvedenko A.G., Shaposhnyk O.A., Kudria I.P., Bublyk O.O. Aging as result of racemic oxymoron, fractal and anti-fractal, Moebius strip like processes. Poltava, ResearchGate, 2018, 75 p.

3. Bartlett G. Systemic thinking: a simple thinking technique for gaining systemic focus. Proceedings of the International Conference on Thinking "Breakthroughs 2001", (www.probsolv.com).

4. Kulishov S.K., Yakovenko O.M., Tretiak N.G. Training for creative thinking as a derivative of system and antisystem comparison, prerequisites for the mathematical modeling. Proceedings of the ICL conference 22.09.- 25.09.2009, the Kassel University Press; 2009, 71-73.

5. Kulishov S.K., Iakovenko O.M., Tretiak N.G. Clinical thinking training as a derivative of system and antisystem comparison, precondition to increase creativity of medical students, physicians. Proceedings of the ICL conference (Hasselt, Belgium) 15.09.-17.09.2010, the Kassel University Press, 2010, 337-343.

6. Bobrov V.A., Kulishov S.K. The adaptive ischemic and reperfusion syndromes in the patients with ischemic heart disease: mechanisms, diagnosis, substantiation of therapy. Dyvosvit, Poltava, 2004, 240 p.

1.2. Multitesting as basis for oxymoron pathology diagnosis as prerequisite to treatment correction

Prerequisite to multitesting of oxymoron like pathology

Audio-video information about using different types of physical, respiratory tests, meditations helped and will help with diagnosis, prophylaxis and treatment oxymoron like pathology. Some authors

[1] demonstrated that multimedia modeling; the neural networks models may be as a basis of prediction course for coronary heart diseases in depression patients and be effective for the establishment of effective treatments and management plans. It's known, "Multimedia Based Clinical Decision Support System for Diagnosis of Chronic Heart Diseases (CHLD-MMCDSS)" gave possibilities to improve the Quality of Life (QOL) of industrial/operational workers suffering from chronic heart diseases and to facilitate diagnosis [2].

The data [3] about multimorbidity, as the manifestation of interconnected networks processes, accentuate significance of multimedia modeling. These processes include genomic, metabolomic, proteomic, and neuroendocrine, immune and mitochondrial bioenergetic elements; social, environmental and health care networks [3]. Stress systems and other physiological mechanisms create feedback loops that integrate and regulate internal networks within the individual [3].

Designing integrative care delivery approaches that more adequately address to the underlying disease processes as the manifestation of a state of physiological disregulation is essential [3].

Purpose of this investigation was using of multimedia modeling of pathogenetic and sanogenetic mechanisms for diagnosis verification, prophylaxis and treatment correction of oxymoron like pathology, including cardiovascular diseases, multimorbidity.

The methodology of multimedia modeling for diagnosis verification, prophylaxis and treatment correction

We proposed and tested algorithm for multimedia modeling of pathogenetic and sanogenetic mechanisms for diagnosis verification, prophylaxis and treatment correction of oxymoron like pathology, icluding cardiovascular diseases, multimorbidity. Object of modeling: diagnosis of disease or diseases, that was or were formulated on the basis of system and antisystem subjective, objective, additional data analysis and their synthesis as oxymoron components [4,5,6].

Model or models for diagnosis verification, prophylaxis and treatment correction of cardiovascular diseases, multimorbidity:

- Hypothesis formulation of the individual pathogenesis, sanogenesis as oxymoron, Moebius strip like [7,8,9,10], fractal and antifractal processes [11,12];
- Determination of some stress-triggers, stress-potentiators, stress-blockators tests as additional investigations program to confirm or to exclude of some mechanisms;
- Structuration, complexation of these research methods, sequence determination of their implementation planning time, as by duration, as by daily time;
- The basis of the complexation of investigations are etiologic, pathogenetic, sanogenetic mechanisms and their relationship each to other;

Approbation of model or models in concrete patient and receiving of the investigation results:

- Multimedia demonstration of investigations program for the patient;
- The repetition of investigation demonstration with parallel their implementation for and by concrete person;

- Evaluation personal additional data by their comparison, making the differential diagnosis decisions.
- Diagnosis verification, prophylaxis and treatment correction.

Additional sub-algorithm for multimedia modeling of oxymoron like heart electrical disturbances mechanisms for ECG conclusion verification, prophylaxis and treatment correction

Object of Modeling: ECG conclusion of rhythm and / or conduction disturbances, that was formulated on the basis of qualitative and quantitative characteristics of ECG waves, segments, intervals by data of usual ECG, Holter ECG monitoring, including results of trigger, potentiator stress tests.

Model or models for ECG conclusion by using:

- hypothesis formulation of the individual heart electrical instability as oxymoron, fractal and antifractal, Moebius strip like processes [7,8,9,10];
- differential geometric analysis of ECG elements rotation bodies - waves, segments, intervals (3D geometry of ECG elements as ellipsoids, cones and others) [12];
- spin direction of rotation waves, segments of ECG [12];
- fractal characteristics of ECG elements (Types of ECG elements by fractal characteristics as Cantor, Koch, Sierpinski sets and others) [11,12];
- antifractal characteristics of ECG elements (Types of ECG elements of antifractal characteristics as anti-snowflake Koch and others) [11,12].
- approbation of ECG model or models in concrete patient and receiving of the investigation results and conclusion formulation;

- ECG conclusion verification, prophylaxis and treatment correction.

Directions of multimedia modeling implementation for diagnosis, prophylaxis and treatment

Implementation of multimedia modeling was based on the complaints, disease history, life history, and data of objective (physical), additional investigations of patients, formulated diagnosis and hypothesis about the individual pathogenesis, treatment plan.

These data, the individual pathogenesis were the basis for the preparation main stream of additional research plan, program with indicating the sequence; the duration of using certain diagnostic methods for diagnosis verification, prophylaxis and treatment correction.

Audio and video of these surveys were collected from investigation internet bank that adds up to concrete patient folder in certain of using sequence.

The physician would present program of some investigations for concrete patient with its multimedia illustration.

This is followed by answers to the questions.

The next step is to conduct research on the type of multimedia material repetition by concrete person and by physician and additional methods control.

As examples of multimedia modeling mechanisms may be presented approaches to patients with various forms of ischemic heart disease in combination with or without neck, thoracic spine osteochondrosis, vertebral artery syndrome, arterial hypertension, chronic obstructive pulmonary disease, bronchial asthma, obliterans atherosclerosis.

Algorithms of sequential, directed to resonating, triggering, potentiating investigations of the pathogenetic and sanogenetic mechanisms, step by step observation of the patients with coronary artery disease combined with arterial hypertension, osteochondrosis and other diseases are presented below.

More concrete examples of multimedia media modeling for diagnosis verification, prescriptions:

- Objects of research are the patients with IHD and osteochondrosis; Methods of investigation – ECG, Holter ECG monitoring. The program of investigation - multimedia model of application sequence of trigger stress tests combination - ECG vertebral test by Ardha Matsyendrasana [13,14], physical exertion by treadmill test or veloergometry.

- Objects of research – the patients with IHD, heart failure and osteochondrosis; Methods of investigation - ECG, Holter ECG monitoring. The program of investigation - multimedia model of application sequence combination of some stress-triggers, potentiators, blockators tests - ECG vertebral test by Ardha Matsyendrasana [13,14], Six Minute Walk Test (6MWT), physical exertion by treadmill test or veloergometry.

- Objects of research – the patients with arterial hypertension; Methods of investigation - ECG, Holter ECG and arterial pressure daily monitoring. The program of investigation - multimedia model of application sequence of stress-triggers, potentiators, blockators tests - veloergometry, pranayama - Single Nostril Breath -Surya Bhedana Pranayama [15], horror movies, emotional and cognitive Stroop test [16], Kumbhaka Pranayama [15], Sitali Breath: Calm Anxiety With Cooling Breath [15].

- Objects of research – the patients with arterial hypertension, hypertensive heart, heart failure; Methods of investigation – ECG, Holter ECG and arterial pressure daily monitoring. The program of investigation - multimedia model of application sequence of stress-triggers, potentiators, blockators tests - horror movies, emotional and cognitive Stroop test [16], pranayama – Bhastrika, "HA" breath to relax [15], veloergometry, Six Minute Walk Test (6MWT)

- Objects of research – the patients with IHD, angina pectoris, stable, II- III functional class, obliterans atherosclerosis; Methods of investigation – ECG, Holter ECG monitoring, vessels Doppler echo. The program of investigation - multimedia model of application sequence of stress tests – veloergometry, hyperventilation test.

The program of patients treatment according to pathogenetic and sanogenetic mechanisms, results of additional investigation included using stress tests for optimization of sanogenetic mechanisms - vertebral asanas, including those, that activation of sinocarotid zone and stellate ganglion; psycho-emotional Stroop test for desensibilization to negativity [16], pranayama by

Bhastrika, Kapalbhati [15], ha-breathing [15]; meditation [17], physical exertion.

Examples of using sub-algorithm of sequential, directed to triggering, resonating, blocking of heart electrical instability investigations, step by step analysis of ECG for making diagnostic decisions are presented below.

Objects of research – usual ECG, Holter ECG monitoring, including results after stress-triggers, stress-potentiators, stress-blockators tests for different cardiovascular pathology, multimorbidity.

Data analysis of ECG conclusion verification has included using of Google 3D modeling program; Autodesk, 3DS MAX, 2015; GeoGebra online and others, hypothesis formulation of the individual heart electrical instability as Moebius strip like processes; rotation bodies of ECG waves, segments, intervals; fractal and antifractal characteristics.

 We have some results of ECG conclusion verification, prophylaxis and treatment correction. Moebius strip like space orientation of depolarization and repolarization processes were characterized by the change of supraventricular pacemaker on ventricular and inverse [7]; by the change of left ventricular pacemaker on right ventricular and inverse; as pair pirouette ventricular premature beats, torsade de pointes ventricular tachycardia. Moebius strip like arrhythmias in the patients with sinus node dysfunction were displayed as a combination of supraventricular and ventricular extrasystoles, fibrillation and flutter transformation from atria to ventricles [7].

The patients with complete atrioventricular block had the Moebius strip like changes of depolarization / repolarization geometry, as the alternation of proximal and distal ventricular rhythms [7].

The specifics of the geometry of depolarization and repolarization processes in the patients with full atrioventricular block or binodal syndrome may be considered in elaborating differential treatment programs to be used in microcomputers for implantable cardiac pacemakers [7].

Analysis of the cardiac depolarization / repolarization geometry may serve as additional criteria for sudden death prognosis [7].

Characteristics of volume, surface, laminar and turbulent data, spin, chirality of rotation bodies of electrocardiogram elements give us possibilities to determine depolarization and repolarization electro-magnetic picture [12], Moebius strip like transitions and iteration, state of electrical heart instabilities [12]. For example, qualitative and quantitative assessment of depolarization-repolarization processes in the patients with complete blockade of the right and / or left bundle branch block allowed to differentiate myocardial infarction, postinfarction cardiosclerosis, and cardiomyopathy [12].

Thus, algorithm of multimedia modeling as basis for making diagnostic decisions of heart electrical instability, including Moebius strip like heart electrical instabilities diagnosis, may be result of qualitative and quantitative, convex, fractal and antifractal characteristics of ECG waves, segments, including ECG elements as bodies of rotation and their spin.

Algorithms of the pathogenetic and sanogenetic mechanisms investigations, observations of the patients with different types of

CHD combined with arterial hypertension, arrhythmias and blockades, heart failure; obliterans atherosclerosis; neck, thoracic osteochondrosis; chronic obstructive pulmonary disease are presented below. Using methods: ECG; Holter ECG monitoring; daily arterial pressure monitoring; spirogram. The program of investigation: multimedia model of application of some stress-triggers, stress-potentiators, stress-blockators tests - hypoxemic; ECG vertebral test by Ardha Matsyendrasana [13,14]; forced vital capacity, forced expiratory volume at 1 second (FEV1), 2 seconds (FEV2), or 3 seconds (FEV3), index of FEV1 divided by FVC; activation sinocarotid zones test; horror movies viewing test; meditation [17]; physical exertion tests.

Conclusion

Thus, algorithm of multimedia modeling for diagnosis verification, prophylaxis and treatment correction of cardiovascular diseases, multimorbidity boils down to the determination of:

- diagnosis of disease or diseases;

- model or models of pathogenetic and sanogenetic mechanisms;

- additional investigations program from combination of some stress-triggers, stress-potentiators, stress-blockators tests;

- approbation of model or models in concrete patient;

- evaluation personal data of investigations;

- diagnosis   verification,   prophylaxis   and   treatment correction.

Referances

1. Junggi Yang, Youngho Lee and Un-Gu Kang. Comparison of Prediction Models for Coronary Heart Diseases in Depression Patients. International Journal of Multimedia and Ubiquitous Engineering,   2015,   10(3):   257-268, http://dx.doi.org/10.14257/ijmue.2015.10.3.24

2. Prem Pal Singh Tomar, Ranjit Singh. Design of Clinical Decision Support System for Chronic Heart Disease Diagnosis Using Case Base Reasoning. Afr J. of Comp & ICTs, 2013, 6(2): 149-160.

3. Sturmberg J.P., Bennett J.M., Martin C.M., Picard M. 'Multimorbidity' as the manifestation of network disturbances. J Eval Clin Pract. 2017 Feb;23(1):199-208. doi: 10.1111/jep.12587. Epub 2016 Jul 15.

4. Kulishov S.K., Yakovenko O.M., Tretiak N.G. Training for creative thinking as a derivative of system and antisystem comparison, prerequisites for the mathematical modeling. Proceedings of the ICL conference 22.09.- 25.09.2009, Villach, Austria, the Kassel University Press, 2009, 71-73.

5. Kulishov S.K., Iakovenko O.M., Tretiak N.G. Clinical thinking training as a derivative of system and antisystem comparison, precondition to increase creativity of medical students, physicians. Proceedings of the ICL conference (Hasselt, Belgium) 15.09.-17.09.2010, the Kassel University Press, 2010, 337-343.

6. Kulishov S.K., Iakovenko O.M. Solving clinical problems using system and anti-system comparison, graphic modeling. INNOVATIVE MEDICINE AND BIOLOGY, Canadian International Monthly Reviewed Journal (CIJIMB), 2011, 3: 30-42.

7. Kulishov S. K., Vorobjov Ye. A, Vakulenko K. Ye., Savchenko A. G., Shevchenko T. I., Latokha I. A. Geometry of depolarization and repolarization processes in IHD patitents of varying age with complete atrioventricular block or binodal disease as precondition to individualized treatment. Problems of aging and longevity, 2006, 15(4): 332-338

8. Kulishov S., Vakulenko K., Latoha I. Myocardial electrical instability as the derivative of inflammation consumption of antiiflammatory factors syndrome, changes in geometry depolarization of atria, ventricles in the patients with coronary heart disease. Absract book of "Rhythm 2011", Congress, Marseile, France, 2011, 39.

9. Kulishov S.K., Vakulenko K.Ye., Iakovenko O.M. Pecularities of cardiac remodeling, cytokines change, electrical myocardial instability in patients with chronic ischemic heart disease and arterial hypertension as predispose to making treatment decision Supplement to Official Journal of the World Heart Federation "Global Heart" (World Congress of Cardiology Scientific Sessions, 2014, Incorporating the Annual Scientific Meeting of the Cardiac Society of Australia and New Zealand), 2014, 9(1S), e 169 (PT 023).

10. Kulishov S.K., Iakovenko O.M. Moebius strip like pathology: mechanisms, diagnosis, treatment correction. Proceedings of the international conference on health informatics and medical

systems (HIMS 2015), ed. H.A. Arabnia, L. Deligiannidis, WORlDCOMP'15, July 27-30, 2015, CSREA Press, 2015, 36-40

11. Kulishov S.K. Genetic algorithm by fractal and anti-fractal exploratory analysis. Clifford Analysis, Clifford Algebras and Their Applications, International Journal; Cambridge Scientific Publishers; 2014, 3(3): 239-248.

12. Kulishov S.K., Iakovenko O.M. Myocardial electrical instability, arterial hypertension as objects for convex and fractal, anti-fractal analysis, optimization of diagnosis. Book of program and abstract of International Conference on Nonlinear Analysis and Convex Analysis,NACA, Chiang Rai, Thailand, (January 21-25, 2015), 2015, 84.

13. Dudchenko M. A., Potiazhenko M.M., Kulishov S.K., Shtepa Iu.A., Khomenko Iu.N. The electrocardiogram characteristics of patients with ischemic heart disease combined with spinal osteochondrosis. Vrachebnoe delo, 1991, 2: 81-84.

14.Kulishov S.K., Tretiak N.G., Kitura O.Ye. Peculiarities of pain, electrocardiogram changes in patients with coronary heart disease and cervical-thoracic osteochondrosis. Medicines of Ukraine, 2007, 2: 35-37.

15. Iyengar B.K.S. The Tree of Yoga. Harper Collins, India; 2005, 208 p.

16.Stroop J.R. Studies of interference in serial verbal reactions. J. Exp. Psychol., 1935, 18: 643–662.

17. O'Doherty V., Carr A., McGrann A., O'Neill J.O., Dinan S., Graham I., Maher V. A controlled evaluation of mindfulness-based

cognitive therapy for patients with coronary heart disease and depression. Mindfulness: 2015; 6(3): 405-416.

1.3. Peculiarities diagnosis of oxymoron like syndromes, diseases, multimorbidity

1.3.1. System and antisystem analysis of syndromes, diseases, multimorbidity as the unity of opposites

Consumption of progredient and antigradient factors: proinflammatory and anti-inflammatory, pro-oxidant and antioxidant, proischemic and anti-ischemic, and others, gave us possibilities to determine syndromes of consumption as basis of multimorbidity [1,2].

The methodology of system and antisystem oxymoron thinking and diagnosis of multimorbidity are presented as a graphical model and program by language "Dragon" – fig. 1,2,3 [1,2,3].

Dragon is visual language, which uses two types of elements: graphic and text labels (inside or outside of graphic shapes) [3]. Operator of the language is graphic element or combination graphic elements together with text labels [3]. Simultaneous use of graphics and text says that the Dragon is addressed not only to the verbal-logical thinking, but activates the intuitive, imaginative thinking [3]. Dragon is not a single language [3]. The family of it includes the hybrid visual programming languages: Dragon-Basic, Dragon-Pascal [3]. Strict separation of visual and textual syntax allows maximum extend the scope of the language, providing it with flexibility and versatility [3].

The methodology of creative system and anti-system oxymoron thinking is presented on visual programming language "Dragon" (fig. 1).

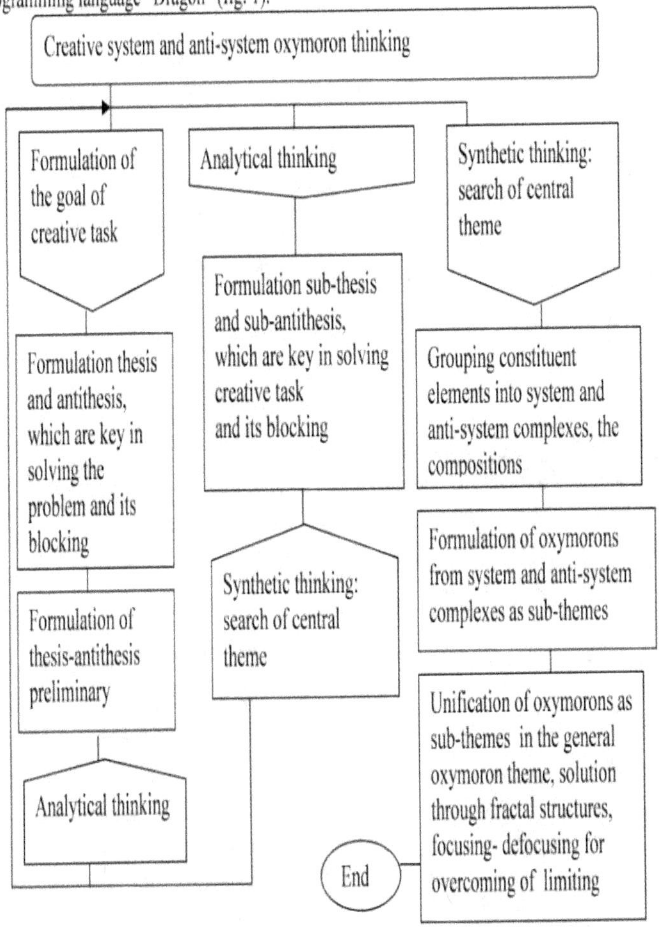

Creative system and anti-system oxymoron thinking

Formulation of the goal of creative task

Analytical thinking

Synthetic thinking: search of central theme

Formulation thesis and antithesis, which are key in solving the problem and its blocking

Formulation sub-thesis and sub-antithesis, which are key in solving creative task and its blocking

Grouping constituent elements into system and anti-system complexes, the compositions

Formulation of thesis-antithesis preliminary

Synthetic thinking: search of central theme

Formulation of oxymorons from system and anti-system complexes as sub-themes

Analytical thinking

Unification of oxymorons as sub-themes in the general oxymoron theme, solution through fractal structures, focusing- defocusing for overcoming of limiting

End

Fig. 1. The methodology of creative system and anti-system oxymoron thinking

Technology of clinical creative thinking, presented as a graphical model and program by language "Dragon" (fig. 2).

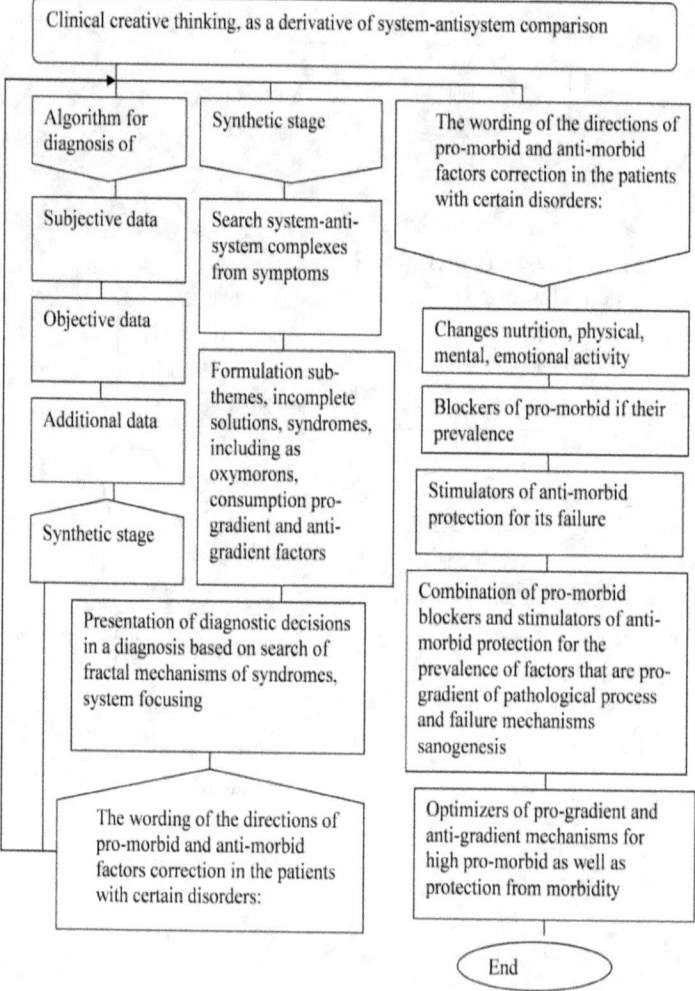

Fig. 2. Algorithm of clinical creative thinking as a graphical model and program by language "Dragon"

Multimorbidity, its mechanisms, triggers is presented on visual programming language "Dragon" (fig. 3).

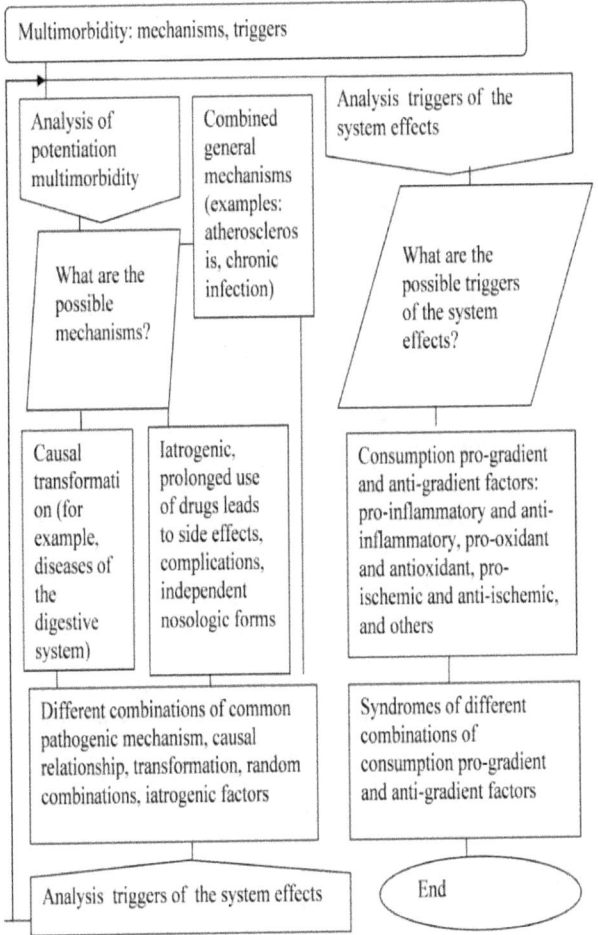

Fig. 3. Multimorbidity, its mechanisms, triggers is presented on visual programming language "Dragon"

Examples of oxymoron complications combination [1]:

- acute renal failure in the patient with chronic renal failure;

- acute respiratory failure in the patient with chronic respiratory failure;

- acute heart failure in the patient with chronic heart failure;

- acute hepatic failure in the patient with chronic hepatic failure (acute poisoning by hepatotoxic compounds in the patient with viral micronodular cirrhosis);

- pro-arrhythmic effects of anti-arrhythmic drugs (amiodarone as trigger of polymorphous ventricular tachycardia);

- pro-ischemic effects of anti-ischemic drugs (steal syndrome by nitroglycerin in the patients with three-vessel coronary artery disease);

- acute atrioventricular block in the patient with chronic atrial fibrillation syndrome.

The following diagnostic algorithm of peripheral arteries remodeling due to consumption of proinflammatory and anti-inflammatory factors [1,4] is presented [1,4]:

- Evaluation of cytokines metabolism;

- Determination of cytokines ratio;

- Determination of carotid, upper and lower extremities arteries remodeling degree;

- Identify the stage of inflammation consumption syndrome (stage I: increase, as pro-inflammatory and anti-inflammatory cytokines with a minimum number of affected arteries; stage II: Increase and decrease some of pro-inflammatory and anti-inflammatory cytokines, inflammatory remodeling of three or four arteries, and more, thickening of intima-media complex from 1 to 1,29 millimetres; stage III: thickening of intima-media complex from 1 to 1.29 millimetres in maximum number of arteries, decrease of both pro-inflammatory and anti-inflammatory cytokines) [1,4].

Examples of oxymoron multisyndromes pathogenesis [1,2]:

- Hypertensive heart disease as set of oxymoron syndromes of pressor and depressor, proinflammatory and anti-inflammatory, prooxidant and antioxidant, stress and antistress, pro-remodeling and anti-remodeling, proarrhythmic and antiarrhythmic processes;

- Acute myocardial infarction as set proishemic and antiischemic, reperfusion and antireperfusion, prooxidant and antioxidant, stress and antistress, proinflammatory and anti-inflammatory, remodeling and antiremodeling, arrhythmic and antiarrhythmic, progradient and antigradient factors of coronary insufficiency.

Emotional intelligence, stress and ischemia, coronary and myocardial failure plays leading roles in progression of ischemic heart disease [5,6]. Older persons with coronary artery disease and concomitant arterial hypertension, and lower ejection fraction were differing by more low level of emotional intelligence [5,6].

Conclusions:

Thus, the proposed technology of solving clinical problems by system and antisystem comparison, presented as a graphical models and programs by languages "Dragon", promotes understanding of complex principles of clinical medicine; improve the quality of diagnosis as precondition to change of the treatment [1].

References

1. Kulishov S.K., Iakovenko O.M. Solving clinical problems using system and anti-system comparison, graphic modeling. J. Innovative Medicine and Biology, 2011, 2-3: 30-42.

2. Bobrov V.A., Kulishov S.K. The adaptive ischemic and reperfusion syndromes in the patients with ischemic heart disease: mechanisms, diagnosis, substantiation of therapy. Dyvosvit, Poltava, 2004, 240 p.

3. Parondzhanov V.D. How to improve the work of the mind. Algorithms without programming - it's easy! M.: Delo, 2001, 360 p.

4. Solomatina L.V., Kulishov S.K. Graphic value of modeling, programming and training in determining vascular remodeling as derivative of arterial pressure's rhythms in patients with hypertension. Proceedings of V international conference "Strategy of quality in industry and education", 4-11 June, 2010; Varna; 2010, 2(1), 617-620.

5.Kulishov S.K., Bublyk O.O. Emotional intelligence in older women with ischemic heart disease in depending on ejection fraction. ResearchGate Publication, The 24th Nordic Congress of Gerontology; Oslo, Norway, 2-4 may 2018 Poster . DOI: 10.13140/RG.2.2.35663.38561

6.Kulishov S.K., Iakovenko O.M., Shvedenko A.G., Shaposhnyk O.A., Kudria I.P., Bublyk O.O. Aging as result of racemic oxymoron, fractal and anti-fractal, Moebius strip like processes. Poltava, ResearchGate, 2018, 75 p.

1.3.2. Diagnosis of oxymoron like peculiarities of heart electrical instabilities

1.3.2.1. System and antisystem analysis of heart arrhythmias and blockades as the unity of opposites, fractal and antifractal antonym pairs

Prerequisites of myocardial electrical instability diagnosis, modeling

Different technologies were used for mathematical modeling of biological rhythms [1,2]. For example, the concept of a contracting excitable medium that is capable of conducting non-linear waves of excitation that in turn initiate contraction [2]. These kinematic deformations have a feedback effect on the excitation properties of the medium [2]. Electrical characteristics resemble basic models of cardiac excitation that have been used to successfully study mechanisms of reentrant cardiac arrhythmias in electrophysiology [2]. It's presenting of a computational framework that employs electromechanical and mechanoelectric feedback to couple a three-variable FitzHugh–Nagumo-type excitation-tension model to the non-linear stress equilibrium equations, which govern large deformation hyperelasticity [2]. Models that describe propagation in the heart generally consist of two parts: a model of the cardiac cell, and a model describing cellular interconnections [2]. Excitation of a cardiac cell is brought about by the change in potential across the cell membrane, due to transmembrane fluxes of various charged ions [2].

It's known that discrimination of electrocardiogram signals using non-linear dynamic parameters is of crucial importance in the cardiac disease therapy and chaos control for arrhythmia defibrillation in the cardiac system [3]. The four nonlinear parameters considered for cardiac arrhythmia classification of the ECG signals are spectral entropy, Poincaré plot geometry, largest

Lyapunov exponent and detrended fluctuation analysis, which are extracted from heart rate signals [3]. Linguistic variables (fuzzy sets) are used to describe ECG features, and fuzzy conditional statements to represent the reasoning knowledge and rules [3].

The methodology of modelling of cardiac arrhythmias and blockades as the unity of opposites, fractal and anti-fractal antonym pairs

Our concept is presented as step by step analysis of electrical myocardial instability. The methodology of this analysis:

- initiation of myocardial electrical instability in concrete case;
- determination of arrhythmic and blockade types;
- searching of disturbance heart rhythm and conductivity components as unity of opposites, antonyms;
- selection of basic and additional antonym pairs;
- conversion of these results as fractal and/ or antifractal antonyms;
- presentation of these data as graphical models by Dragon language [4].

Conversion of cardiac arrhythmias and blockades as fractal and/ or antifractal antonyms by genetic algorithm [5,6,7,8] promote understanding of arrhythmogenesis, triggers and resonators of these processes; improve the quality of diagnosis as precondition to correct treatment. Genetic algorithm may be as fractal and /or antifractal producing machine. We take a pairs of chromosomes, consisting from fractals and/ or anti-fractals. Chromosome genes may be sets and anti-sets: Cantor, Julia, Mandelbrot, von Koch, Sierpinski carpet, Peano curve, Peano anti-curve, the Hilbert curve, Darer pentagon, Cantor square, tricorn and multicorns. As a result of crossing-over (one-, two-point or multi-point), we get new offspring chromosomes consisting from different combinations of genes. Results of modeling of cardiac arrhythmias and blockades as the unity of opposites, fractal and antifractal antonyms are presented on language Dragon [4] (fig. 1).

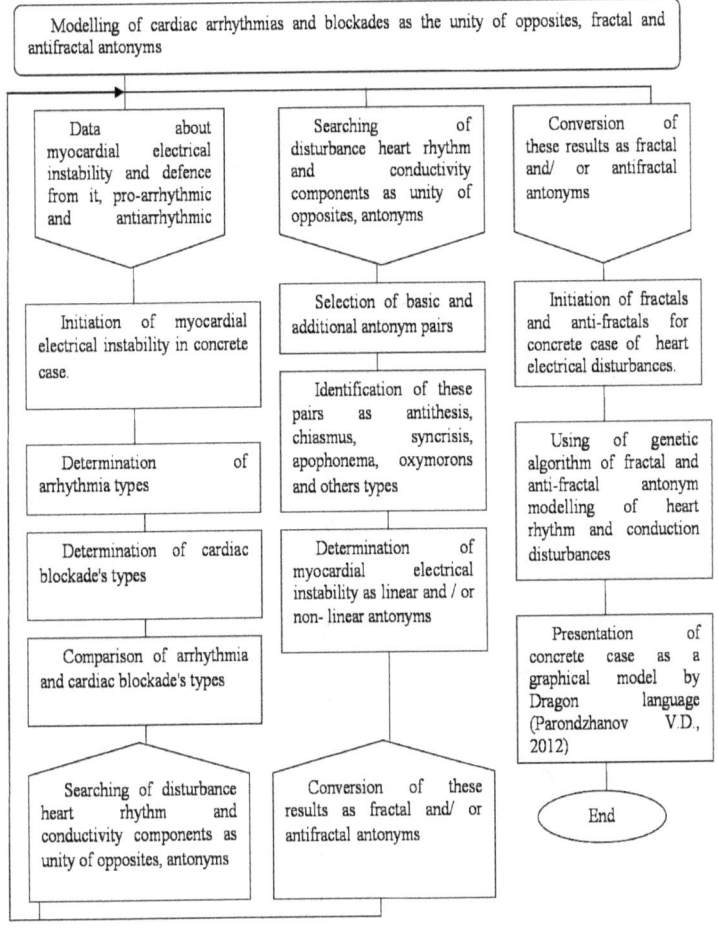

Fig. 1. Modelling of cardiac arrhythmias and blockades as the unity of opposites, fractal and antifractal antonyms

Genetic algorithm of fractal and anti-fractal antonym modeling of heart rhythm and conduction disturbances is presented on language   Dragon   [4] (fig.2).

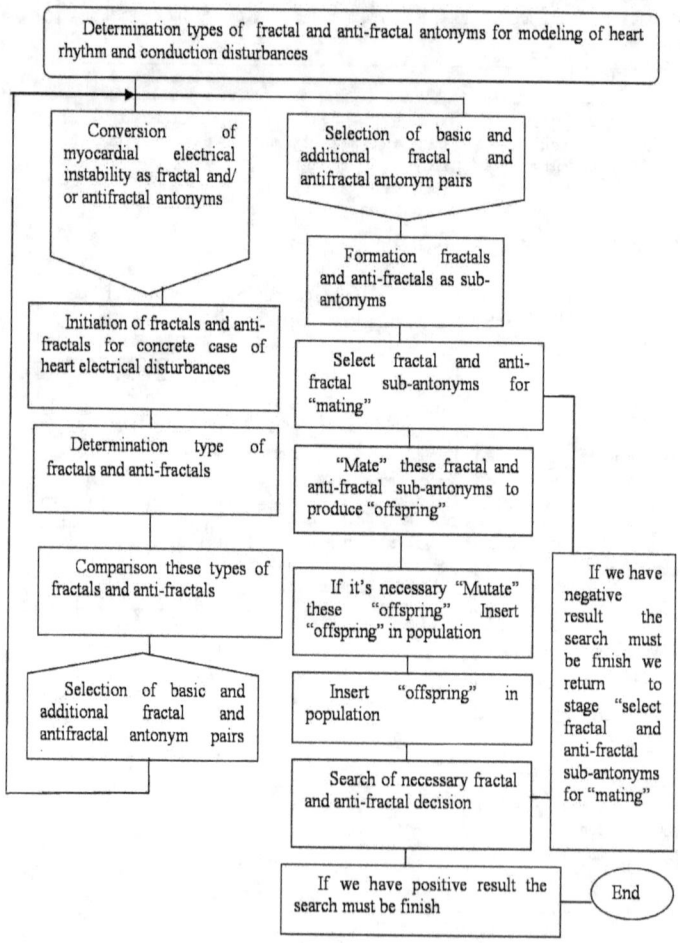

Fig. 2. Genetic algorithm of fractal and anti-fractal antonym modelling of heart rhythm and conduction disturbances

Implementation of modeling of cardiac arrhythmias and blockades as the unity of opposites, fractal and antifractal antonym pairs

Diagnosis mechanisms of oxymoron like heart electrical instabilities by different parameters

Examples of linear and nonlinear antonym pathogenesis of heart arrhythmias and blockades as result of unity:

- Sinus node dysfunction as sinoatrial blockade II stage and atrial fibrillation;

- Sinus node dysfunction as tachycardia-bradycardia syndrome: bradycardia may originate in the sinus node, atria, atrioventricular junction, or ventricle; the tachycardia is caused by atrial flutter or fibrillation, reentrant supraventricular tachycardia;

- Binodal syndrome as sinus node dysfunction and atrioventricular node block;

- Trifascicular block - right bundle branch with both left anterior fascicular and left posterior fascicular, and atrioventricular III block.

Examples of heart electrical instabilities oxymoron pathogenesis as result of unity:

- Mechanisms of left ventricular extrasystole: excitation of left ventricular with functional block of right bundle-branch;

- Mechanisms of right ventricular extrasystole: excitation of right ventricular with functional block of left bundle-branch.

Examples of oxymoron heart electrical instabilities by orientation of depolarization and repolarization processes:

- The Moebius strip like space orientation of depolarization processes were characterized by the change of supraventricular pacemaker and ectopic activity onto the ventricular one;

- In the patients with sick sinus syndrome, the Moebius strip like arrhythmias were displayed as a combination of supraventricular and ventricular extrasystoles, pair fibrillation and flutter transformation from atria to ventricles;

- The patients with complete atrioventricular block showed the Moebius strip like changes of depolarization and repolarization geometry as the alternation of proximal and distal ventricular rhythms [9].

Electrical instability of the heart is derived from structural and electrical remodeling [9,10,11].

Rhythm and conduction disturbances may be represented by various known fractals and anti-fractals. Examples of fractal and anti-fractal mechanisms of oxymoron like heart electrical instabilities:

Thesis - arrhythmia as fractals (triggers);

Antithesis - conduction disturbance of the heart as antifractals (resonators);

Oxymoron - sum of heart rhythm and conduction disturbances as triggers and resonators.

We may have inverse variant:

Thesis: conduction disturbance of the heart as fractals (triggers);

Antithesis: arrhythmia as antifractals (resonators);

Oxymoron: sum of triggers and resonators of heart electrical instabilities.

Different types of heart electrical instabilities as oxymorons by time and heart space parameters:

Thesis - Paroxysmal atrial fibrillation;

Antithesis - Constant intra-atrial blockage;

Oxymoron - sum of paroxysmal atrial fibrillation and constant intra-atrial blockage.

Different types of heart electrical instability as oxymorons by morphological disturbances degree:

Thesis - functional and organic arrhythmia;

Antithesis - functional and organic conduction disturbance;

Oxymoron - sum of functional and organic arrhythmia, functional and organic conduction disturbance.

Next example:

Thesis - functional arrhythmia;

Antithesis - organic conduction disturbance;

Oxymoron - sum of functional arrhythmia, organic conduction disturbance.

Some others variants of heart electrical instabilities combination:

Thesis - functional and organic arrhythmia;

Antithesis - organic conduction disturbance;

Oxymoron - sum of functional and organic arrhythmia, organic conduction disturbance.

And:

Thesis - functional and organic arrhythmia;

Antithesis - functional conduction disturbance;

Oxymoron - sum of functional and organic arrhythmia, functional conduction disturbance.

And:

Thesis - functional arrhythmia;

Antithesis - functional and organic conduction disturbance;

Oxymoron - sum of functional arrhythmia, functional and organic conduction disturbance.

And:

Thesis - organic arrhythmia;

Antithesis - functional and organic conduction disturbance;

Oxymoron - sum of organic arrhythmia, functional and organic conduction disturbance.

And:

Thesis - organic arrhythmia;

Antithesis - functional conduction disturbance;

Oxymoron - sum of organic arrhythmia, functional conduction disturbance.

And:

Thesis - organic arrhythmia;

Antithesis - organic conduction disturbance;

Oxymoron - sum of organic arrhythmia, organic conduction disturbance.

And:

Thesis - functional arrhythmia;

Antithesis - functional conduction disturbance;

Oxymoron - sum of functional arrhythmia and functional conduction disturbance.

Bradyarrhythmias as oxymoron like heart rhythm and conduction disorders. Different types of sinus node dysfunction as automaticity, contractility, conductibility and excitability oxymorons:

Basis of our creative ECG solving method is necessary to compare the elements systems and antisystems as rate, rhythm, charactestics of P waves, PR (PQ) interval, Q waves, R waves, S waves, T waves, U waves, J waves, QRS complex, QT interval, ST segment for diagnosis binodal syndrome (disease). The algorithm consists from:

- Formulation thesis (or antithesis), which are key in solving the problem of determination of heart conduction disturbances, presence of sum sinoatrial node disfunction and atrioventricular blockade data;

- Formulation of antithesis the presence of arrhythmia, including atrial fibrillation, supraventricular and ventricular tachycardia, tachycardia-bradycardia syndrome and others;

- Introduction thesis and antithesis as combination of preliminary oxymorons-solutions. Oxymorons are a proper subset of the expressions called contradictions in presence combination of different heart conduction and rhythm disturbances.

Example:

Thesis - Sinoatrial blockage II stage;

Antithesis - Atrial fibrillation;

Oxymoron - Sick sinus syndrome as sinoatrial blockage II stage and atrial fibrillation.

Different types of fascicular blockages as conductibility oxymorons:

Examples:

Thesis - left anterior fascicular block;

Antithesis - left posterior fascicular block;

Oxymoron - both left anterior fascicular block and left posterior fascicular block is equal left bundle branch block.

And:

Thesis - left bundle branch block;

Antithesis - right bundle branch block;

Oxymoron - both left and right bundle branch block.

And:

Thesis - right bundle branch block;

Antithesis - left anterior fascicular block;

Oxymoron - bifascicular block - right bundle branch block with left anterior fascicular block.

And:

Thesis - right bundle branch block;

Antithesis - left posterior fascicular block;

Oxymoron - bifascicular block - right bundle branch block with left posterior fascicular block.

Tachyarrhythmias as oxymoron like heart rhythm and conduction disorders

Example:

Thesis - WPW syndrome;

Antithesis - functional block of usual (normal) conduction system (pathway);

Oxymoron - mechanisms of WPW syndrome: impulse is conducted on additional pathway with functional block of usual (normal) conduction system.

Different types of heart activities as contractility, conductibility and excitability oxymorons:

Examples:

- Pair racemic, pirouette ventricular extrasystoles as sum of left ventricular and right ventricular extrasystoles;

- Sum of the ventricular and supraventricular extrasystoles (pair of ventricular and supraventricular extrasystoles) as Moebius strip like arrhythmia; substitutive rhythms;

Example:

Thesis - left atrial extrasystoles accompanied by a functional blockade of right atrium;

Antithesis - right atrial extrasystoles accompanied by a functional block of left atrium;

Oxymoron - Multifocal atrial tachycardia.

Diagnosis of oxymoron like heart electrical instabilities as prerequisite for prognosis of disease course and treatment correction

The specifics of the geometry of depolarization and repolarization processes may be as prerequisite for treatment correction, prognosis of disease course:

- Analysis of the cardiac depolarization and repolarization geometry may serve as additional criteria for sudden death prognosis [9].

- The specifics of the geometry of depolarization and repolarization processes in the patients with full atrioventricular block and binodal disease can be considered in elaborating differential treatment programs for implantable cardiac pacemakers [9].

Heart electrical instabilities as fractals and antifractals

Heart rhythm and conduction disturbances can be represented by various known fractals and antifractals. Genetic algorithm for fractal, antifractal modeling of the heart rhythm and conduction disorders reduced to the formation of population, each person which is a chromosome, which reflects a certain type of myocardial electric instability. Each chromosome consists from genes, where each gene is a certain fractal, antifractal element of atrial and ventricular depolarization and repolarization changes. The criteria for selection and evaluation of its results is conformity the spatial organization of the electromagnetic processes as a combination of fractals, antifractals with certain spin, chirality and structural, electrical remodeling of the heart. If it's necessary, we use the operator of mutations to improve modeling of pathogenic mechanisms, fractal and antifractal foundations of the heart rhythm and conduction disorders, myocardial electrical instability. The goal of making optimization and modeling decision is to achieve a compiling of individual fractal and/ or antifractal combination that were selected models of cardiac structural and electrical disturbances.

So Sierpinski napkin may reflect small and large sclerotic processes in the myocardium, as a result of coronary artery disease (fig. 3). At the same time, this kind of fractal and Cantor set may reflect multiple foci of atrial depolarization during atrial fibrillation. Koch set may be a prototype, model of CLC, WPW syndromes; left, right bundle branch blockades. Tricorn and multicorns antifractals can be a model of re-entry effect.

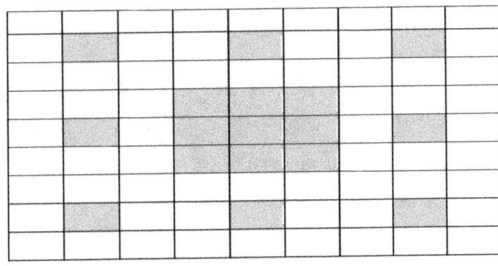

Fig. 3. Small and large sclerotic processes in the myocardium by coronary artery disease as the "carpet" Sierpinski

Dissemination and the concentration of the excitation wave on the myocardium can be represented as a set and anti-Cantor set (fig. 4).

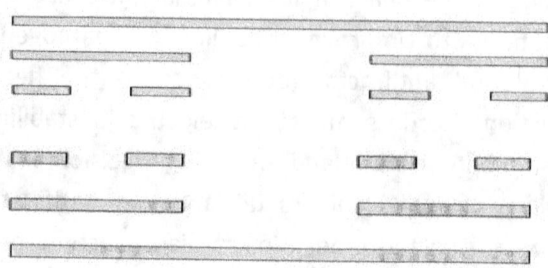

Fig. 4. Dissemination and the concentration of the excitation wave on the myocardium as a set and anti-Cantor set

Conclusion

Thus, the proposed technology of making electrical myocardial instability diagnosis decisions by system and antisystem comparison, formation fractal and antifractal cardiac arrhythmic and blockade antonym pairs.

Proposed algorithms, graphical models promote understanding of arrhythmogenesis, triggers and resonators of these processes; improve the quality of diagnosis as precondition to correct treatment.

Referances

1. Glass L., Mackey M.C. From Clocks to Chaos: The Rhythms of Life. Princeton University Press, 1988, 248 pp.

2. Nash M.P., Panfilov A.V. Electromechanical model of excitable tissue to study reentrant cardiac arrhythmias. Progress in Biophysics and Molecular Biology, 2004, 85(2-3):501-522.

3. Anuradha B., Veera Reddy V.C. Cardiac arrhythmia classification using fuzzy classifiers. Journal of Theoretical and Applied Information Technology, © 2005 - 2008 JATIT, 353-359.

4. Parondzhanov V.D. How to improve the work of the mind. Algorithms without programming - it's easy! M.: Delo, 2001, 360 p.

5. Bobyryov V. M., Kulishov S.K., Vakhnenko A. V., Vlasova O.V. Genetic algorithm for making pharmacotherapy decision in the patients with multimorbidity. Wiad Lek, 2017; 71, 6 cz. I: 1142-1145

6.Kulishov S.K. Genetic algorithm by fractal and anti-fractal exploratory analysis. Clifford Analysis, Clifford Algebras and Their Applications, 2014; 3(3): 239-248.

7.Kulishov S.K., Iakovenko O.M.: The combination of on-line and off-line learning of genetic algorithm application in diagnostic and therapeutic decision making in internal medicine clinic. Proceedings of the ninth international conference "New Information Technologies in Education for All", 2014, 25-26 November, Ukraine, Kyiv, 2014, 287-291.

8. Kulishov S.K., Iakovenko O.M., Shvedenko A.G., Shaposhnyk O.A., Kudria I.P., Bublyk O.O. Aging as result of racemic oxymoron, fractal and anti-fractal, Moebius strip like processes. - Poltava, ResearchGate, 2018, 75.

9. Kulishov S. K., Vorobjov Ye. A, Vakulenko K. Ye., Savchenko A. G., Shevchenko T. I., Latokha I. A. Geometry of depolarization and repolarization processes in IHD patitents of varying age with complete atrioventricular block or binodal disease as precondition

to individualized treatment "Problems of aging and longevity ", 2006, 15, № 4. - P. 332-338

10. Kulishov S., Vakulenko K., Latoha I. "Myocardial electrical instability as the derivative of inflammation consumption of antiiflammatory factors syndrome, changes in geometry depolarization of atria, ventricles in the patients with coronary heart disease", Absract book of "Rhythm 2011", Congress, Marseile, France, 2011, p. 39.

11. Kulishov S.K., Vakulenko K.Ye., Iakovenko O.M. Fractal and antifractal analysis of triggers and resonators in electrical instability in the patients with coronary heart disease and sinus node dysfunction // Supplement to Official Journal of the World Heart Federation "Global Heart" (World Congress of Cardiology Scientific Sessions, 2014, Incorporating the Annual Scientific Meeting of the Cardiac Society of Australia and New Zealand), 2014, March, Vol. 9, Issue 1S, e 169 (PT 022).

1.3.2.2. Graph theory, convex analysis as basis for diagnosis of oxymoron like heart electrical Instabilities

Prerequisites for analysis and modeling of oxymoron like heart electrical instability

Mathematics [1,2,3,4,5,6], including graph theory [1], topology [3,5,6], convex analysis [2,4] have been studied and applied to medicine, cardiology [3,4]. Heart electrical instability has various causes. The differential diagnosis of it is based on qualitative and quantitative electrocardiogram assessment.

The purpose of this study was to formulate an algorithm for making diagnosis of heart electrical instability as oxymoron, fractal and anti-fractal, Moebius strip like processes by using discrete mathematics, graph theory, topology, convex analysis, multiple testing.

Methodology of oxymoron like heart electrical instability analysis and modeling

We used algorithm for diagnosing heart electrical instability, which reduces to qualitative and quantitative analysis of ECG in standard, inverted, 3D (as rotation bodies of ECG's elements) forms (Autodesk, 3DS MAX, 2015); constructing graphs, including "Gift wrapping" algorithm; calculation distances between points, angles between graphs, and others; comparison of qualitative and quantitative characteristics of these graphs by selective multiple testing [7]; formulation of the diagnostic conclusion.

Implementation of making diagnosis decisions by oxymoron like heart electrical instability analysis and modeling

Characteristics of volume, surface, laminar and turbulent data, spin, chirality of rotation bodies of electrocardiogram elements give us possibilities to determine depolarization and repolarization electro-magnetic picture, oxymoron, fractal and anti-fractal, Moebius strip like transitions and iteration, state of electrical heart instabilities [8,9].

Examples:

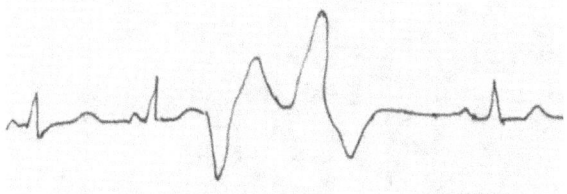

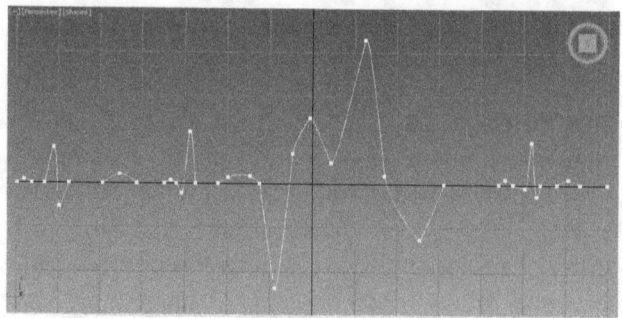

Fig. 1. Pair pirouette ventricular premature (example 1)

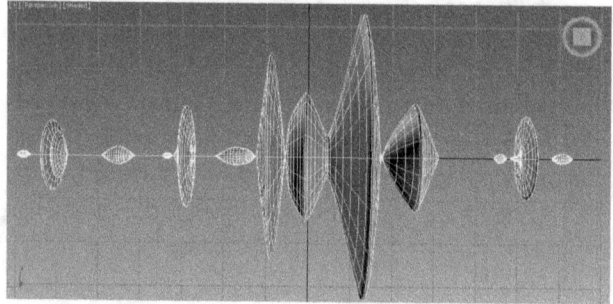

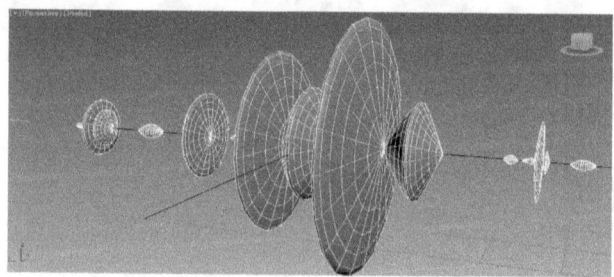

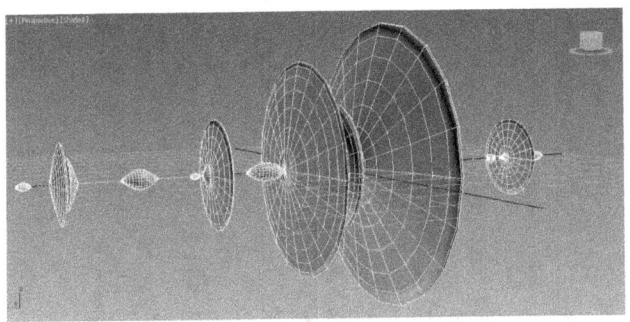

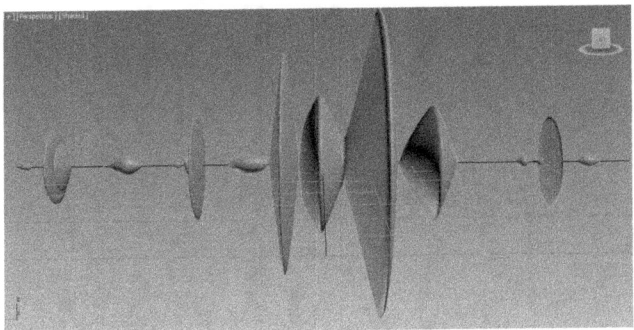

Fig. 2. Rotation bodies of electrocardiogram elements in the patient with pair pirouette ventricular premature beats (example 1)

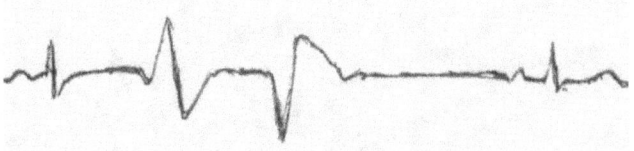

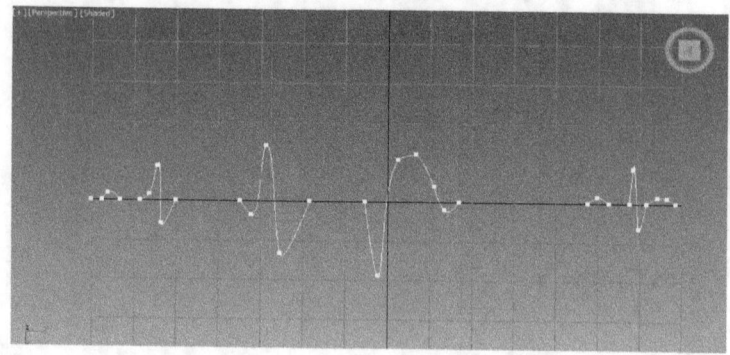

Fig. 3. Pair pirouette ventricular premature (example 2) [8,9]

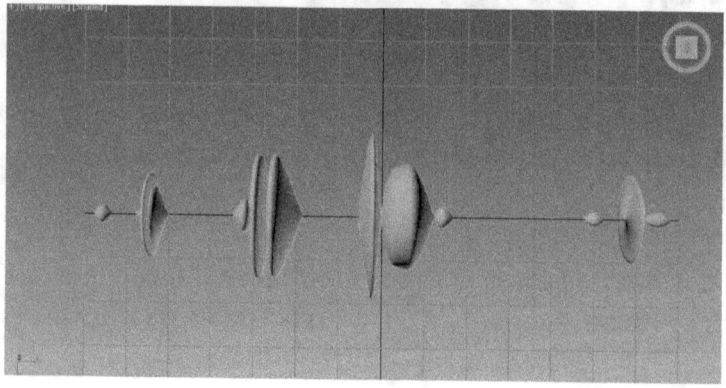

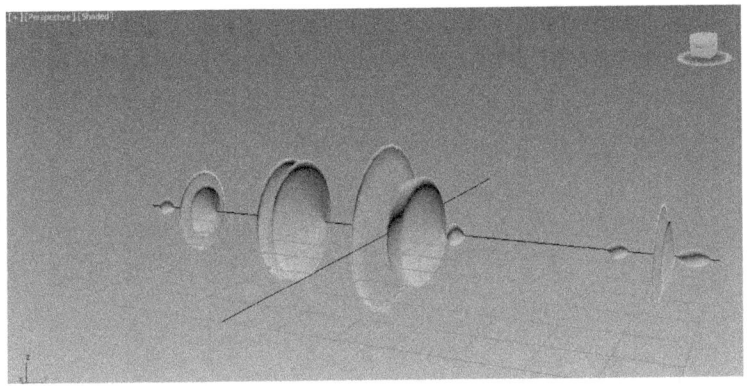

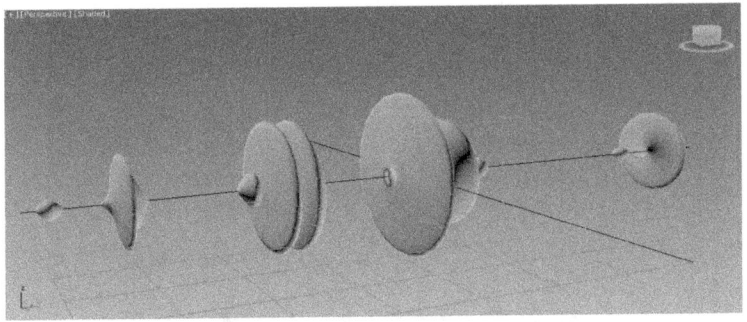

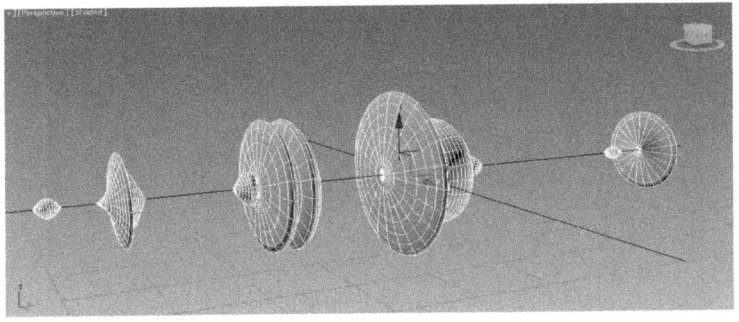

Fig. 4. Rotation bodies of electrocardiogram elements in the patient with pair pirouette ventricular premature beats (example 2)

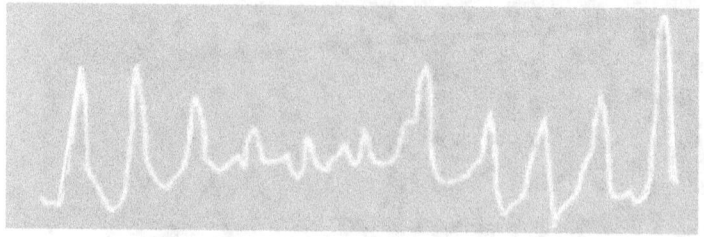

Fig. 5. Torsade de pointes ventricular tachycardia

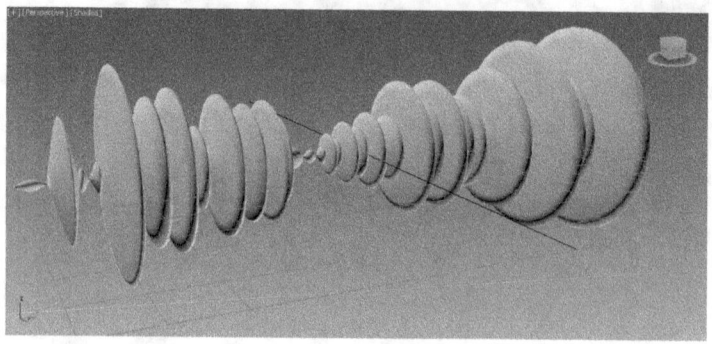

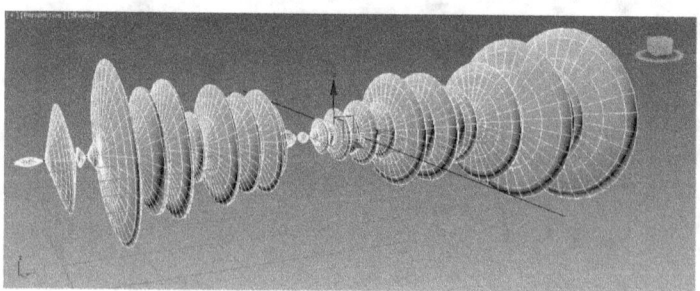

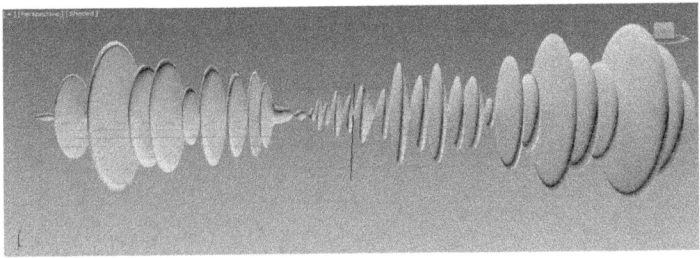

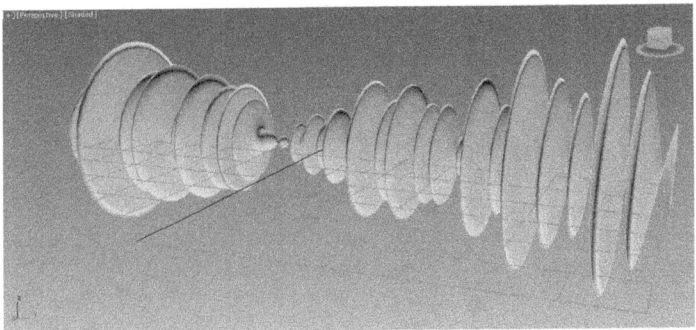

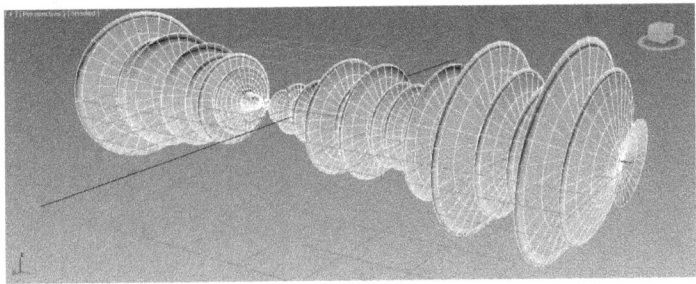

Fig. 6. Rotation bodies of electrocardiogram elements in the patient with torsade de pointes ventricular tachycardia

Principles of electrocardiogram analysis by construction of the convex hull, by "Gift wrapping" algorithm for determination the relationship between the investigated PQSRT elements are presented by example (fig. 7):

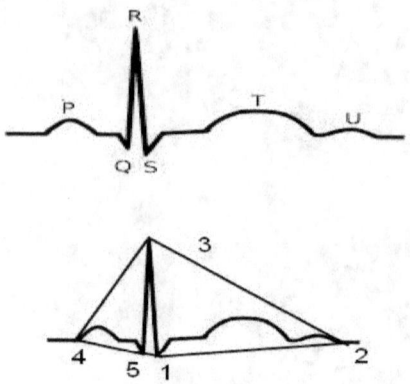

Fig. 8. Joining of PQSRT complex points according to "Gift wrapping" algorithm

Construction of the convex hull for determination the relationship between the investigated electrocardiogram complexes as Moebius strip like constituents in the patients with pair pirouette ventricular premature beats (fig. 9).

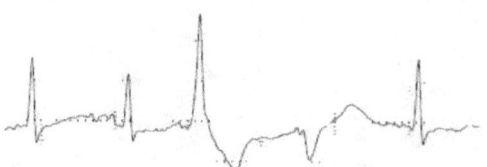

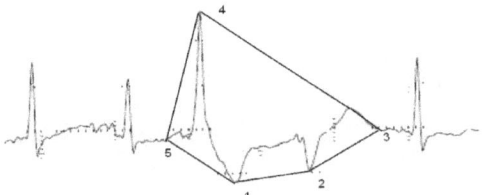

Fig. 9. The convex hull of ECG complexes as Moebius strip like constituents in the patients with pair pirouette ventricular premature beats

Construction of the convex hull for determination the relationship between the investigated ECG elements as Moebius strip like constituents in the patients with torsade de pointes ventricular tachycardia (fig. 10).

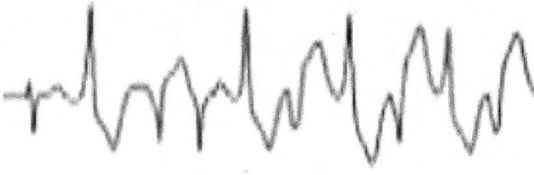

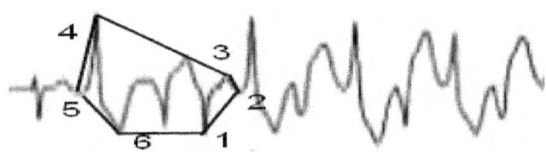

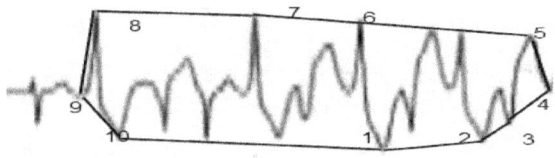

Sergii K. Kulishov

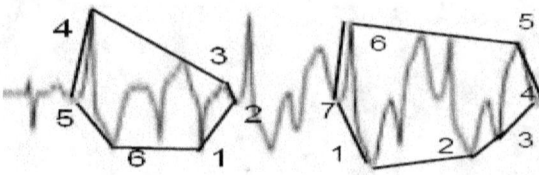

Fig. 11. The convex hull of ECG complexes as Moebius strip like constituents in the patients with torsade de pointes ventricular tachycardia

Investigating of "Gift wrapping" algorithm for ECG gave us possibilities to use these curves as for convex analysis and as for graph building of heart electrical network instabilities mechanisms.

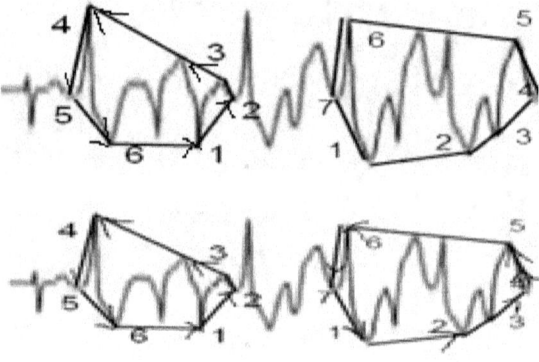

Fig. 12. The convex hull of ECG complexes as Moebius strip like constituents in the patients with torsade de pointes ventricular tachycardia

Construction of the convex layers for determination the relationship between the investigated complexes as Moebius strip like constituents in the patients with torsade de pointes ventricular tachycardia (fig. 13,14).

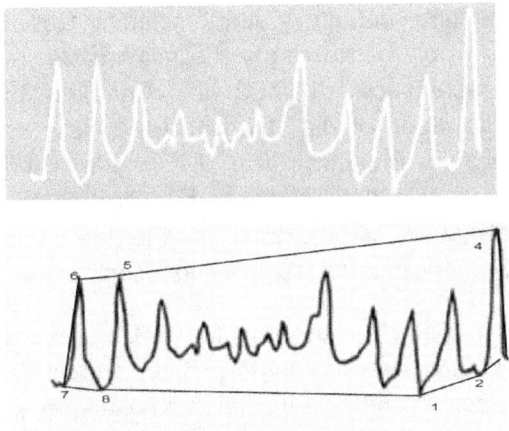

Fig. 13. The convex layers of ECG complexes as Moebius strip like constituents in the patients with torsade de pointes ventricular tachycardia

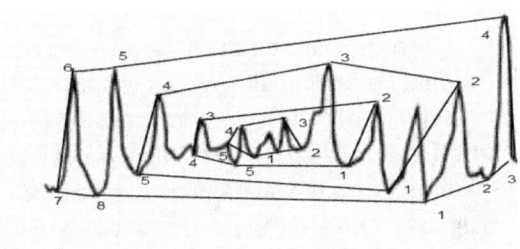

Fig. 14. The convex multiply layers of ECG complexes as Moebius strip like constituents in the patients with torsade de pointes ventricular tachycardia

Characteristics of electrocardiogram by type, distance between points, perimeters, angles of polygons of complexes allowed to determine depolarization and repolarization electromagnetic picture, triggers and resonators of Moebius strip like electrical heart instabilities.

The construction of indefinite, definite graphs, including closed and open graphs, made it possible to clarify the mechanisms of arrhythmogenesis. Characteristics of ECG by chirality of depolarization and repolarization of the atria and ventricles, the presence of oxymoron and Moebius strip like rhythm and conduction disorders, their spin data, distance between points, perimeters, angles of polygons of complexes allowed to determine peculiarities of electromagnetic picture, triggers and resonators.

Investigating of "Gift wrapping" algorithm for ECG gave us possibilities to use these curves as for convex analysis and as for graph building of heart electrical network instabilities mechanisms.

Changes of electrocardiogram complexes, intervals in the patients with myocardial electrical instabilities give us some types and sizes rotation figures as complexes from ellipsoid, sphere, cone and others figures.

Conclusions

Thus, complex using of discrete mathematics, graph theory, topology, convex analysis, multiple testing allowed us to formulate an algorithm for making diagnosis of heart electrical instability as oxymoron, fractal and anti-fractal, Moebius strip like processes. Analysis of graphs as networks of node-waves with their ribs will improve the quality of diagnosis and treatment the patients with heart rhythm and conduction disorders.

References

1.Basavaprasad B., Ravindra S. Hegadi   A graph theoretical network model of human heart.   International J. of Applied Engineering Research, 2014, 9 (20): 4549-4552.

2.Chazele Bernand On the convex layers of a plenar set. IEE Transactions on information theory, 1985, it-31 (4), 509-510.

3.Kulishov S.K., Iakovenko O.M. Fractal and antifractal oxymorons, Moebius strip like transformations of biomedical data as basis for exploratory subgroup analysis. Book of abstract of International Conference on Trends and Perspective in Linear Statistical Inference; LinStat, (2014), Linkoping, Sweden, 2014, 24-28.

4.Kulishov S.K., Iakovenko O.M. Myocardial electrical instability, arterial hypertension as objects for convex and fractal, anti-fractal analysis, optimization of diagnosis. Book of program and abstract of International Conference on Nonlinear Analysis and Convex Analysis (NACA 2015, Chiang Rai, Thailand, January 21-25, 2015), 2015, 84.

5.Kulishov S.K., Iakovenko O.M. Moebius strip like pathology: mechanisms, diagnosis, treatment correction. Proceedings of the 2015 international conference on health informatics and medical systems (HIMS 2015), ed. H.A. Arabnia, L. Deligiannidis, WORlDCOMP'15, Las Vegas, USA. (July 27-30, 2015), CSREA Press, 2015, 36-40.

6.Kulishov S., Vakulenko K., Latoha I. Myocardial electrical instability as the derivative of inflammation consumption of antiiflammatory factors syndrome, changes in geometry depolarization of atria, ventricles in the patients with coronary heart disease. Absract book of "Rhythm 2011" Congress, Marseille, France, (May 26-28 2011), 2011, 39.

7.Kulishov S.K. Creative solutions as derivatives of selective multiple testing, Booklet. CIRM conference: Mathematical Methods of Modern Statistics; Luminy; (10-14th July 2017), 2017, 21-22.

8.Kulishov S.K., Iakovenko, O.M. Shvedenko, A.G. Convex Analysis of Age Dependent Heart Electrical Instability. ResearchGate

Publication, The 24th Nordic Congress of Gerontology; Oslo, Norway, 2-4 may 2018, Poster. DOI: 10.13140/RG.2.2.12175.28325

9.Kulishov S.K., Iakovenko O.M., Shvedenko A.G., Shaposhnyk O.A., Kudria I.P., Bublyk O.O. Aging as result of racemic oxymoron, fractal and anti-fractal, Moebius strip like processes. Poltava, ResearchGate, 2018, 75 p.

1.4. Aging and age dependent diseases as a deriving of genes expressing, racemic oxymoron, fractal and antifractal processes

1.4.1. Aging as result of racemic oxymoron, fractal and antifractal processes

Aging theory algorithm may be formulated as result of [1,2,3]:

- Racemic oxymoron, fractal and antifractal, Moebius strip like processes;

- Activation and inhibition of telomerase, deoxyribonucleic acid;

- Reducing the synergy between the human genome and the genome of skin and intestinal microorganisms.

Examples of oxymoron pathogenesis of diseases, aging and the anti-aging racemic processes [1,2,3]:

Arterial hypertension is a set of oxymoron syndromes of pro-inflammatory and anti-inflammatory [1,2,3], pro-oxidant [1,2,3] and antioxidant [1,2,3], stress and anti-stress [1,2,3], pro-remodeling and anti-remodeling [1,2,3], pro-arrhythmic and antiarrhythmic [1,2,3] processes;

Acute myocardial infarction as a set pro-ischemic and anti-ischemic [1,2,3], stress and anti-stress [1,2,3], pro-inflammatory [1,2,3] and anti-inflammatory [1,2,3], remodeling and anti-remodeling [1,2,3], arrhythmic and antiarrhythmic [1,2,3], pro-gradient [1,2,3] and anti-gradient [1,2,3] factors of coronary insufficiency.

Examples of oxymoron pathogenesis of arrhythmias: The Moebius like space orientation of depolarization processes were characterized by the change of supraventricular pacemaker and ectopic activity onto the ventricular one [1,2,3].

In the patients with sick sinus syndrome, the Moebius like arrhythmias [1,2,3] were displayed as a combination of supraventricular and ventricular extrasystoles, pair fibrillation and flutter transformation from atria to ventricles [1,2,3]. The patients with complete atrioventricular block showed the Moebius like changes of depolarization and repolarization geometry as the alternation of proximal and distal ventricular rhythms [1,2,3].

Conclusion

Aging as result of racemic oxymoron, fractal and antifractal, Moebius strip like processes was proposed on the basis of own and others authors investigations.

References

1. Kulishov S.K., Iakovenko O.M. Aging as result of racemic oxymoron, fractal and anti-fractal, Moebius strip like processes. Programme, 2-4 may 2018 LESSONS OF A LIFETIME Oslo 24 NKG 2018 (24th Nordic Congress of Gerontology); 2018, 127.

2. Kulishov S.K., Iakovenko O.M. Aging as result of racemic oxymoron, fractal and anti-fractal, Moebius strip like processes. ResearchGate Publication, The 24th Nordic Congress of Gerontology; Oslo, Norway, 2-4 may 2018, Poster. DOI: 10.13140/RG.2.2.13853.00484

3. Kulishov S.K., Iakovenko O.M., Shvedenko A.G., Shaposhnyk O.A., Kudria I.P., Bublyk O.O. Aging as result of racemic oxymoron, fractal and anti-fractal, Moebius strip like processes. Poltava, ResearchGate, 2018, 75 p.

1.4.2. Monitoring of age dependent diseases as a reflection of aging genes expressing, racemic oxymoron, fractal and antifractal processes

Prerequisites for analysis and modeling of aging dynamics

Ageing is one of the most important and relevant topics of all mankind [1,2]. In the last years there has been an intensive search for candidates for the role of genes of death and longevity in humans [1,2,3]. In view of the large number of candidate genes involved in aging, is now the focus is on the genes that are homologous to genes determining longevity in animals of other species, and genes responsible for the development of the main diseases associated with aging [1,2].

Establishing genetic features longevity and determination of the genetic status of key genes involved in the pathogenesis of age-dependent diseases, are the main approaches to the identification of the key components of active aging and longevity [1,2].

Candidate genes participate in the processes of aging can be classified as [1,2]:

• involving in maintaining the balance of cell tissues (apoptosis genes, telomerase);

• control the integrity of the genome and DNA repair;

• determine resistance to stress (heat shock genes, and antioxidant protection);

- cause epigenetic changes (methylation, carbonylation and nitrosylation).

Recently, it was found that oxidative stress (excessive formation of reactive oxygen species - ROS) can significantly accelerate the shortening of telomeres and is an integral part of cellular aging, as well as exacerbating pathologies characteristic of old age [1,2]. To neutralize ROS in the cell there is a system of antioxidant protection [1,2]. Repression or overexpression of antioxidant enzyme genes significantly alters life expectancy [1,2]. One of the key enzymes of this system is superoxide dismutase (MnSOD, SOD2) [1,2,4]. At various model organisms MnSOD was demonstrated influence on aging and longevity [1,2]. There are data on the association of gene polymorphism SOD2 (SOD2-9T / C) with the development of pathologies seniors: atherosclerosis, hypertension, cardiomyopathy, diabetic nephropathy, some cancers, etc. [1,2,5]

Anti-aging medicine is a medical specialty founded on the application of advanced scientific and medical technologies for the early detection, prevention, treatment, and reversal of age-related dysfunction, disorders, and diseases [1,2]. It is a healthcare model promoting innovative science and research to prolong the healthy lifespan in humans [1,2]. As such, anti-aging medicine is based on principles of sound and responsible medical care that are consistent with those applied in other preventive health specialties [1,2].

Medical science has cataloged many signs of senescence [1,2,3]. It manifests as dozens of changes in cells, tissues, and organs during aging [1,2]. Human life is supported by a complex network of biochemical substances and reactions which affect the physical state and vitality of the body and mind [1,2]. Senescent changes can be seen in the rate and outcome of many of these reactions [1,2,3]. However, many of these changes are secondary effects of senescence, rather than primary causes [1,2,3]. Chronic inflammation is a well-known corollary of the aging process and is believed to significantly contribute to morbidity and mortality of many age-associated chronic diseases [1,2,4]. However, the mechanisms that cause age-associated inflammatory changes are not well understood [1,2]. Particularly, the contribution of cell stress responses to age-associated inflammation in 'non-inflammatory' cells remains poorly defined [1,2,4].

Chronic inflammation associated with the aging process has been implicated in a host of degenerative disease states including osteoarthritis, atherosclerosis, 2nd type diabetes [1,2]. Age-associated chronic inflammatory states are distinct from inflammation triggered by infection [1,2,3]. It is presently unclear to what extent chronic inflammatory states in older individuals represent autoimmune processes caused by deregulation of the immune system [1,2,4]. Alternatively, these states may arise as a consequence of an increased cell stress response in old cells triggered by molecular damage incurred over a lifetime [1,2].

We consider that analysis of age dependent diseases manifestations, as a reflection of genes expressing, help us to determine rhythms of aging and antiaging process, its possible mechanisms [1,2]. Monitoring of age dependent diseases manifestations by sensors of motion, registration of electrocardiograms (ECGs), electromyograms (EMGs), electro-encephalograms (EEGs), respiratory rhythm, glycemic level may be basis for this analysis [1,2]. It's known that the emerging m-Health concept represents the evolution of e-health systems loosely defined as the use of the Internet for healthcare to mobile applications without guaranteed Internet connectivity [1,2,5]. The advances in m-Health systems are driven by the developments in wireless communications, pervasive, and wearable technologies [1,2,5]. A typical Wireless Body Area Network (WBAN) consists of a number of inexpensive, lightweight, and miniature sensor platforms, each featuring one or more physiological sensors, e.g. motion sensors, ECGs, EMGs, EEGs [1,2,5]. The sensors could be located on the body as tiny intelligent patches, integrated into clothing, or implanted below the skin or muscles [1,2,5].

The purpose of this work is solving problem of age dependent diseases monitoring as a reflection of aging genes expressing using system and anti-system comparison, graphic modeling, programming, exploratory analysis on the principles of Cantor, von Koch sets, Cantor square fractal and anti-fractal concepts [1,2].

The methodology of analysis and modeling age diseases monitoring as a reflection of aging genes expressing

Algorithm of system and anti-system comparison for solving clinical problems of age dependent diseases monitoring as a reflection of aging genes expressing boils down to [1,2]:

- The formation of the pro-aging and anti-aging factors set;

- Formulation sub-thesis and sub-antithesis, which are key in solving creative task and its blocking;

- Formulation of preliminary solution of this task;

- Grouping constituent elements into system and anti-system complexes, the compositions;

- Formulation of oxymorons from system and anti-system complexes as sub-themes;

- Unification of oxymorons as sub-themes in the general oxymoron theme, solution through fractal structures, focusing- defocusing for overcoming of limiting search of central theme the transformation of intermediate preliminary solution in the final decisions.

The methodologies of fractal data transformation for exploratory statistical analysis have 3 steps [1,2,6].

The first step is [1,2,6]:

•   selection of informative numerical dependent variabilities for transformation to categorical types by using Cantor, von Koch or others sets principles as basis, triggers for exploratory clinical research analysis.

The second step is statistical analysis of these informative numerical variabilities [1,2,6]:

•   Determination of mean, standard error of mean, standard deviation, 95% confidence interval for mean, median, minimum, maximum, range, quartiles, interquartile range, skewness, kurtosis.

•   Determination of the variabilities distribution - parametric or nonparametric by single-factor the Kolmogorov-Smirnov test; Shapiro-Wilk W test and graphical methods: frequency distribution histograms stem & leaf plots; scatter plots; box & whisker plots; normal probability plots: PP and QQ plots; graphs with error bars (Graphs: Error Bar).

The third step is [1,2,6,7]:

•   To choose using Cantor or von Koch sets principles for transformation informative numerical variabilities to categorical types by results of statistical analysis. More high level of standard deviation, interquartile range is better for using Cantor or von Koch sets principles. Algorithm of exploratory data analysis using the technology of the iteration process as for receiving Cantor set [4,5]:

•   Selection of informative numerical dependent variabilities;

•   Transformation these informative numerical dependent variabilities to categorical variabilities;

•   Formation categorical variabilities in the form of subgroups with the maximum, median and minimum values;

• Formation of a new categorical variabilities in the form of sub-subgroups with maximum, median and minimum values in the subgroups with the highest and lowest values (closed ring);

• Formation categorical variabilities in the form of subgroups as a result of an iterative process as for Cantor set;

• Statistical analysis of the data;

• Determination of the variabilities distribution - parametric or nonparametric by single-factor the Kolmogorov-Smirnov test; Shapiro-Wilk W test and graphical methods: frequency distribution histograms stem & leaf plots; scatter plots; box & whisker plots; normal probability plots: PP and QQ plots; graphs with error bars (Graphs: Error Bar);

• Transformations that may be normalize of non-normality data: If residuals have a right skew, should apply a square-, a cube- or fourth-root, a logarithmic, and an inverse transformation to data. If residuals have a left skew, should raise to the second, third or fourth power, an exponential transformation to data;

• ANOVA - Analysis of Variance, with variations depending on the linear nature of variability. Method of multiple comparison groups Tukey HSD, Scheffe, Bonferroni if deviations were homogeneous for the test Levene, and in the absence of homogen eity - the criteria Tamhane's T2, Games-Howell;

• Nonparametric equivalent of ANOVA / MANOVA - Kruskal-Wallis test;

• Formulation of a conclusion based on statistical analysis.The methodologies of other fractal and anti-fractal data transformation for exploratory statistical analysis have basis of different iterative process.

Summary data of analysis and modeling age diseases monitoring as a reflection of aging genes expressing [1,2]

Algorithm of rhythms and fractals aging and anti-aging diagnosis is reduced to the determination of the episodes of maximum and minimum or without manifestations of age-dependent pathology [1,2]. Age-dependent pathology, as the expression of genes of aging, is presented by the symptoms, syndromes, diseases, multimorbidity states, more often the cardiovascular, respiratory, endocrine, digestive and nervous systems [1,2]. Triggers of the aging process are the effects of anti-aging factors consumption [1,2]. Monitoring the activity of internal organs allows to evaluate the dynamics of these processes [1,2].

Algorithm for diagnosis of aging rhythms and fractals is reduced to the determination the episodes of [1,2]:

• Small range of diurnal changes of the heart rate (chronotropic insufficiency);

• The appearance of disturbances of rhythm and conduction from minimum to maximum, life dangerous level;

• Arterial hypertensive or hypotensive reactivity, increasing arterial pulse pressure;

• Hypopnea or apnea during the night;

• Syndrome "restless legs" at night;

• Hypoglycemia, hyperglycemia;

• Desynchronosis of cardiovascular, respiratory, glycemia, hormonal rhythms. The mechanisms that favor the appearance of aging fractals on the gene, the subcellular (including the mitochondrial level), cellular, tissue, organ, system, organism as a whole are:

• Syndromes of consumption of aging progradient and antigradient, pro-morbidity and anti-morbidity, pro-oxidant and anti-oxidant, pro-inflammatory and anti-inflammatory, pro-ischemic and anti-ischemic, pro-arrhythmic and anti-arrhythmic, and other factors;

• Changes of the cardiovascular, brain, skeletal muscle electromagnetic processes in space and time, as Moebius strip;

• Changes of cardiovascular, respiratory, glycemia, hormonal rhythms similar to those known in the climate effects, as El Nino and La Nina;

• The transition from mono- to multimorbidity;

• Narrowing of chaotic influences that lead to aging and anti-aging disbalance.

Algorithm of anti-aging rhythms and fractals is reduced to the determination [1,2] of various episodes of synchronization of rhythms in the range of the golden section, Fibonacci numbers, the lack of activation of the above signs of age-dependent pathology. Increasing of duration of the age-dependent pathology deactivation determines adaptation to aging and reflects decreased expression of genes of aging [1,2].

Examples of the results of the algorithm for using principles of Cantor set for Exploratory Data Analysis of clinical research data [1,2] are presented by determination of the dependence between tolerance to stress, inflammation syndrome, coronary and myocardial failure, arterial pressure, ventricular arrhythmias in the patients with coronary heart disease and essential hypertension [8,9,10,11,12,13].

Fractal analysis of monitoring glycemic profile and arterial pressure helped with diagnosis of the sum negative effects in the patients with 1st diabetes mellitus in combination with essential hypertension [1,2,14]. Daily changes in glucose levels, blood pressure, heart rate are the basis of individual diagnosis of pathogenic mechanisms, the correction of the treatment of the patients with diabetes mellitus in combination with essential hypertension [1,2,14].

Additional studies may clarify the mechanisms of aging and the role of [1,2,3]:

- Oxidation, glycation, cross-linking, and other chemical modifications all act to impair the molecular functioning of multiple vital components, including DNA, membranes, the extracellular matrix (ECM), enzymes, and structural proteins. Modifications which accumulate faster than they are repaired or recycled will cause progressive deterioration over time;

- Junk molecules and aggregates accumulate inside and outside of cells;

- The redox potential poise of some cells changes in response to these chemical modifications. This results in altered gene expression, altered enzyme activity, and altered signaling pathways;

- Repair and recycling mechanisms slow down;

- A minority of deteriorating cells release chemicals which harm other, healthy cells;

- The neuroendocrine and immune systems seem to follow a developmental program of decline, which may cause them to send chemical signals of differentiation and death to various tissues;

- Cells are lost by apoptosis and necrosis, especially among nondividing cells of the heart, skeletal muscle, and brain substantia nigra. Organs and tissues deteriorate over time when cells are lost faster than they are replaced;

- Stem cells stop dividing and no longer replace.

New perspective additional studies may clarify the mechanisms of aging and the role of [1,2,15] the sinus node as the primary pacemaker of the heart [1,2,15]. A complex interplay of heterogeneities is assumed to be the basic mechanism that the sinus node can drive the heart. This interplay can be disturbed by e.g. diseases, drugs or mutations. In this work the effect of a mutation on the sinus node function were investigated [1,2,15]. Therefore, measurement data of wild-type and mutant I Kr channels were integrated with aid of optimization procedures into the heterogeneous sinus node model [1,2,15] The measurement data shows a shift of the steady state inactivation to more positive potentials [1,2,15]. Simulated central sinus node cells lose their ability to depolarize spontaneously [1,2,15]. Peripheral cell are also effected by the mutation [1,2,15]. The main changes are the shortening of the action potential duration from 108 ms to 84 ms and the increase of auto-rhythmic frequency from 6.37 Hz to 7.62 Hz due to an increased mean I Kr current. In a future study the bradycardia effect of this mutation will be shown in a tissue model [1,2,15].

Solution of the age dependent pathology monitoring as a reflection of aging gene expression is reduced to the determination of the ratio of gradient and anti-gradient fractals by exploratory system and anti-system analysis, synthesis [1,2]. This algorithm is a system of operations to convert data in the result as a generalized solution [1,2]. The presence of efficient algorithms for solving problems which are before, contributes to a positive outcome [1,2].

Conclusion. Our algorithm system and anti-system comparison, graphic modeling, programming, exploratory analysis on the principles of Cantor, von Koch sets, Cantor square fractal and anti-fractal concepts will help maximize insight, uncover underlying structure, extract important variables, develop models and determine optimal factor settings, may improve possibilities of diagnosis and treatment, body and genome nets building [1,2].

References

1. Kulishov S.K., Iakovenko O.M. Modeling Monitoring Of Age Dependent Diseases as a Reflection Of Aging Genes Expressing. International Journal of Modeling and Optimization (IJMO), IACSIT (International Association of Computer Science and Information Technology), Singapore, 2013, 3(1),: 25-29.

2. Kulishov S.K., Iakovenko O.M., Shvedenko A.G., Shaposhnyk O.A., Kudria I.P., Bublyk O.O. Aging as result of racemic oxymoron, fractal and anti-fractal, Moebius strip like processes. - Poltava, ResearchGate, 2018, 75 p.

3. Vijg J. Aging of the Genome: The Dual Role of DNA in Life and Death. New York, USA: Oxford University Press Inc.; 2007, 384 p.

4. Kriete A. Biomarkers of aging: combinatorial or system model? Sci Aging Knowledge Environ.; 2006, (1): pe1.

5. Jovanov E. Wireless technology and system integration in body area networks for m-health applications. In Proceedings of the 27th Annual International Conference of the IEEE Engineering in Medicine and Biology Society, 2005.

6.Kulishov S.K., Iakovenko O.M. Fractals as triggers exploratory statistical analysis of clinical pharmacological data, International journal of pharmacology and pharmaceutical technology (IJPPT), 2012, 1(1): 53-57.

7. Shaver C. An Exploration of the Cantor Set. Rockhurst University .09, James and Elizabeth Monahan Summer Research Fellowship, Summer 2008, MT4960: Mathematics Seminar, Spring, 2009, 19 p.

8.Bobrov V.O., Kulishov S.K. The adaptive ischemic and reperfusion syndromes in the patients with ischemic heart disease: mechanisms, diagnosis, substantiation of therapy. Poltava: Dyvosvit, 2004, 240.

9.Kulishov S.K., Iakovenko O.M. Solving clinical problems using system and anti-system comparison, graphic modeling. Innovative Medicine and Biology, Canadian International Monthly Reviewed Journal (CIJIMB), 2011, 3: 30-42.

10.Kulishov S., Kudria I. Stress and inflammation as determinative factors in the patients with coronary heart disease and essential hypertension. Final programme& Abstract Book of the European Conference. 2nd edition "Heart, Vessels & Diabetes", 3-5 November, Athens, Greece, 2011, 50

11.Kulishov S., Vakulenko K., Latoha I. Myocardial electrical instability as the derivative of inflammation consumption of antiiflammatory factors syndrome, changes in geometry depolarization of atria, ventricles in the patients with coronary heart disease. Absract book of "Rhythm 2011," Congress, Marseile, France, 2011, 39.

12. Kulishov S. K., Kudria I.P., Vakulenko K.Ye. Method of diagnosis of circadian stress and stress-limitative rhythms in patients with ischemic heart disease in combination with essential hypertension. The patent of Ukraine for utility model no. 41598 IPC (2009) A 61 B 5/02, , 2009, Bulletin No 10.

13. Kulishov S. K., Vakulenko K.Ye. Method of diagnosis of systemic disturbances of desynchronosis of arterial pressure, respiratory, cardiac rhythms. The patent of Ukraine for utility model no. 41598 IPC (2009) A 61 B 5/02; A 61 B 5/0205, 2009, Bulletin No 12, 2009.

14.Kulishov S., Iakovenko O. Individual diagnostic value of monitoring blood glucose and arterial pressure in the patients with diabetes mellitus and essential hypertension: a case report. Final programme& Abstract Book of the European Conference. IInd edition "Heart, Vessels & Diabetes", no. 3-5, Athens, Greece, 2011, 51.

15. Seemann G., Scholz Ep., Weiss Dl., Dossel O. Effects of the Reggae Mutations on Synus Node Function: A Simulation Study. Computers in Cardiology, 2008, 35: 421-424.

Chapter 2. Principles of oxymoron like pathology treatment correction

2.1. Fractals as triggers for exploratory statistical analysis of clinical pharmacological data

Prerequisites of fractal and antifractal data transformation as the basis, triggers for exploratory statistical analysis [1]

The essence of good prescribing is to pick the most appropriate drug for the disease in question, taking pathophysiology in account [1,2,3]. Drugs act on a wide variety of targets: receptors, transport processes, enzymes, by others miscellaneous effects [1,2,3]. Following administration, disposition of drugs in the body is determined by drug absorption, distribution, metabolism and excretion [1,2,3]. Taken together, these processes define pharmacokinetics of drug [1,2]. Drug therapy monitoring, also known as Therapeutic Drug Monitoring (TDM), is a means of monitoring drug levels in the blood [1,2,3]. Because so many different factors influence blood drug levels, the following points should be taken into consideration during TDM: the age and weight of the patient; the route of administration of the drug; the drug's absorption rate, excretion rate, delivery rate, and dosage; other medications the patient is taking; other diseases the patient has; the patient's compliance regarding the drug treatment regimen; and the laboratory methods used to test for the drug [1,2,3]. TDM is a practical tool that can help the physician provide effective and safe drug therapy in patients who need medication [1,2,3]. Monitoring can be used to confirm a blood drug concentration level that is above or below the therapeutic range, or if the desired therapeutic effect of the drug is not as expected [1,2]. If this is the case, and dosages beyond normal then have to be prescribed, TDM can minimize the time that elapses [1,2,3].

TDM is important for patients who have other diseases that can affect drug levels, or who take other medicines that may affect drug levels by interacting with the drug being tested [1,2,3]. Therapeutic drug monitoring refers to the individualization of dosage by maintaining plasma or blood drug concentrations within a target range (therapeutic range, therapeutic window) [1,2,3]. There are two major sources of variability between individual patients in drug response [1,2,3]. These are variation in the relationship between: dose and plasma concentration (pharmacokinetic variability); drug concentration at the receptor and the response (pharmacodynamic variability) [1,2,3]. Several methods have been developed to improve the prediction of individual dose requirements based on sparse data for individual patients [1,2,3]. These are based either on calculation of clearance and volume of distribution from one or a few timed drug concentrations, or by a Bayesian feedback method [1,2,3]. This latter method is based on differences between 'typical' population parameter values and those predicted for the individual patient from measured drug concentrations [1,2,3].

Exploratory Data Analysis (EDA) is an approach/philosophy for data analysis that employs a variety of techniques (mostly graphical) to [1,2]:

- maximize insight into a data set;

- uncover underlying structure;

- extract important variables;

- detect outliers and anomalies;

- test underlying assumptions;

- develop parsimonious models;

- determine optimal factor settings.

Most EDA techniques are graphical in nature with a few quantitative techniques [1,2]. The reason for the heavy reliance on graphics is that by its very nature the main role of EDA is to open-mindedly explore, and graphics gives the analysts unparalleled power to do so, enticing the data to reveal its structural secrets, and being always ready to gain some new, often unsuspected, insight into the data [1,2]. In combination with the natural pattern-recognition capabilities that we all possess, graphics provides, of course, unparalleled power to carry this out [1,2].

For classical analysis, the sequence is from problem to data, model, analysis, conclusions [1,2].

For EDA, the sequence is from problem to data, analysis, model, conclusions [1,2]. For Bayesian, the sequence is problem, data, model, prior distribution, analysis, conclusions [1,2].

Thus for classical analysis, the data collection is followed by the imposition of a model (normality, linearity, etc.) and the analysis, estimation, and testing that follows are focused on the parameters of that model [1,2]. For EDA, the data collection is not followed by a model imposition; rather it is followed immediately by analysis with a goal of inferring what model would be appropriate [1,2]. Finally, for a Bayesian analysis, the analyst attempts to incorporate scientific/engineering knowledge/expertise into the analysis by imposing a data-independent distribution on the parameters of the selected model; the analysis thus consists of formally combining both the prior distribution on the parameters and the collected data to jointly make inferences and/or test assumptions about the model parameters [1,2].

The classical approach imposes models (both deterministic and probabilistic) on the data [1,2]. Deterministic models include, for example, regression models and analysis of variance (ANOVA) models [1,2]. The most common probabilistic model assumes that the errors about the deterministic model are normally distributed-this assumption affects the validity of the ANOVA F tests [1,2].

The Exploratory Data Analysis approach does not impose deterministic or probabilistic models on the data. On the contrary, the EDA approach allows the data to suggest admissible models that best fit the data [1,2].

The two approaches differ substantially in focus. For classical analysis, the focus is on the model - estimating parameters of the model and generating predicted values from the model [1,2].

For exploratory data analysis, the focus is on the data - its structure, outliers, and models suggested by the data [1,2].

Classical techniques are generally quantitative in nature. They include ANOVA, t tests, chi-squared tests, and F tests [1,2].

EDA techniques are generally graphical. They include scatter plots, character plots, box plots, histograms, bihistograms, probability plots, residual plots, and mean plots [1,2].

Classical estimation techniques have the characteristic of taking all of the data and mapping the data into a few numbers ("estimates") [1,2]. This is both a virtue and a vice. The virtue is that these few numbers focus on important characteristics (location, variation, etc.) [1,2]. The vice is that concentrating on these few characteristics can filter out other characteristics (skewness, tail length, autocorrelation, etc.) of the same population [1,2]. In this sense there is a loss of information due to this "filtering" process [1,2].

The purpose of this work is using Cantor, von Koch sets principles as basis, triggers of exploratory clinical research analysis for better insight into a data [1,2].

The methodology of fractal data transformation for exploratory statistical analysis [1,2]

The methodologies of fractal data transformation for exploratory statistical analysis have 3 steps [1,2]. The first step is [1,2]:

- selection of informative numerical dependent variabilities for transformation to categorical types by using Cantor, von Koch or others sets principles as basis, triggers for exploratory clinical research analysis.

Cantor set obtained from the closed interval from 0 to 1 by removing the middle third from the interval, then the middle third from each of the two remaining sets, and continuing the process indefinitely [1,2,4]. The Cantor ternary set is created by repeatedly deleting the open middle thirds of a set of line segments. One starts by deleting the open middle third (1⁄3, 2⁄3) from the interval [0, 1], leaving two line segments: [0, 1⁄3] ∪ [2⁄3, 1] [1]. Next, the open middle third of each of these remaining segments is deleted, leaving four line segments: [0, 1⁄9] ∪ [2⁄9, 1⁄3] ∪ [2⁄3, 7⁄9] ∪ [8⁄9, 1] [1,2,4]. This process is continued ad infinitum. The Cantor set cannot contain any interval of non-zero length [1,2,4]. In fact, it may seem surprising that there should be anything left — after all, the sum of the lengths of the removed intervals is equal to the length of the original interval [1,2]. However, a closer look at the process reveals that there must be something left, since removing the "middle third" of each interval involved removing open sets (sets that do not include their endpoints) [1]. So removing the line segment (1/3, 2/3) from the original interval [0, 1] leaves behind the points 1/3 and 2/3 [1]. Subsequent steps do not remove these (or other) endpoints, since the intervals removed are always internal to the intervals remaining [1,2,4].

The second step is statistical analysis of these informative numerical variabilities [1,2]:

- Determination of mean, standard error of mean, standard deviation, 95% confidence interval for mean, median, minimum, maximum, range, quartiles, interquartile range, skewness, kurtosis.

- Determination of the variabilities distribution - parametric or nonparametric by single-factor the Kolmogorov-Smirnov test; Shapiro-Wilk W test and graphical methods: frequency distribution histograms stem & leaf plots; scatter plots; box & whisker plots; normal probability plots: PP and QQ plots; graphs with error bars (Graphs: Error Bar).

The third step is [1,2]:

- To choose using Cantor or von Koch sets principles for transformation informative numerical variabilities to categorical types by results of statistical analysis. More high level of standard deviation, interquartile range is better for using Cantor or von Koch sets principles.

Algorithm of exploratory data analysis using the technology of the iteration process as for receiving Cantor set [1,2]:

- Selection of informative numerical dependent variabilities;

- Transformation these informative numerical dependent variabilities to categorical variabilities;

- Formation categorical variabilities in the form of subgroups with the maximum, median and minimum values;

- Formation of a new categorical variabilities in the form of sub-subgroups with maximum, median and minimum values in the subgroups with the highest and lowest values (closed ring);

- Formation categorical variabilities in the form of subgroups as a result of an iterative process as for Cantor set;

- Statistical analysis of the data;

- Determination of the variabilities distribution - parametric or nonparametric by single-factor the Kolmogorov-Smirnov test; Shapiro-Wilk W test and graphical methods: frequency distribution histograms stem & leaf plots; scatter plots; box & whisker plots; normal probability plots: PP and QQ plots; graphs with error bars (Graphs: Error Bar);

- Transformations that may be normalize of non-normality data: If residuals have a right skew, should apply a square-, a cube- or fourth-root, a logarithmic, and an inverse transformation to data. If residuals have a left skew, should raise to the second, third or fourth power, an exponential transformation to data;

- ANOVA - Analysis of Variance, with variations depending on the linear nature of variability. Method of multiple comparison groups Tukey HSD, Scheffe, Bonferroni if deviations were homogeneous for the test Levene, and in the absence of homogeneity - the criteria Tamhane's T2, Games-Howell;

- Nonparametric equivalent of ANOVA / MANOVA - Kruskal-Wallis test;

- Formulation of a conclusion based on statistical analysis.

Algorithm of exploratory data analysis using the technology of the iteration process as for receiving von Koch set [1,2]:

- Selection of informative numerical dependent variabilities;

- Transformation these informative numerical dependent variabilities to categorical variabilities;

- Formation categorical variabilities in the form of subgroups with the maximum, median and minimum values;

- Formation of a new categorical variabilities in the form of sub-subgroups with maximum and minimum values in the subgroup with median values (closed ring);

- Formation categorical variabilities in the form of subgroups as a result of an iterative process as for von Koch set;

- Statistical analysis of the data;

- Determination of the variabilities distribution - parametric or nonparametric by single-factor the Kolmogorov-Smirnov test; Shapiro-Wilk W test and graphical methods: frequency distribution histograms stem & leaf plots; scatter plots; box & whisker plots; normal probability plots: PP and QQ plots; graphs with error bars (Graphs: Error Bar);

- Transformations that may be normalize of non-normality data: If residuals have a right skew, should apply a square-, a cube- or fourth-root, a logarithmic, and an inverse transformation to data. If residuals have a left skew, should raise to the second, third or fourth power, an exponential transformation to data;

- ANOVA - Analysis of Variance, with variations depending on the linear nature of variability. Method of multiple comparison groups Tukey HSD, Scheffe, Bonferroni if deviations were homogeneous for the test Levene, and in the absence of homogeneity - the criteria Tamhane's T2, Games-Howell;

- Nonparametric equivalent of ANOVA / MANOVA - Kruskal-Wallis test;

- Formulation of a conclusion based on statistical analysis.

Some illustrations of graphic modeling, programming of using fractal transformation of data as the basis for exploratory statistical analysis [1,2]

Examples of the results of the algorithm for using principles of Cantor, von Koch sets for Exploratory Data Analysis of clinical research data [1,2] are presented by syndromes of the consumption as a common biological principle of desadaptation and diagnosis of the viable, stunned, hibernation myocardium and cardiac protective precondition on the basis of modeling of biochemical, instrumental, mathematical, coronary-ventricular data [5,6,7,8,9].

Examples of the results of the algorithm for using principles of Cantor set for Exploratory Data Analysis of clinical research data are presented by determination of the dependence between tolerance to stress, inflammation syndrome, coronary and myocardial failure, arterial pressure, ventricular arrhythmias in the patients with coronary heart disease and essential hypertension [1,2,10,11].

Fractal analysis of monitoring glycemic profile and arterial pressure helped with diagnosis of the sum negative effects in the patients with 1st diabetes mellitus in combination with essential hypertension [1,2,12]. Daily changes in glucose levels, blood pressure, heart rate are the basis of individual diagnosis of pathogenic mechanisms, the correction of the treatment of the patients with diabetes mellitus in combination with essential hypertension [1,2,12].

Transformations of variables may be by recode and compute procedures [1,2]. The recode procedure is typically used with transformations involving categorical variables [1,2]. It is the best option when we want to create a categorical distinction based on an existing numeric variable [1,2]. Using the technologies of the iteration process as for receiving Cantor, von Koch or others sets for transformations of variables may be by recode procedure [1,2]. If new variables that consist from subgroups similar as the Cantor, von Koch or others sets will have non-normal distribution we use the compute procedure [1,2]. This procedure allows the analyst to perform mathematical operations on variables [1,2].

References

1. Kulishov S.K., Iakovenko O.M. Fractals as triggers exploratory statistical analysis of clinical pharmacological data. International journal of pharmacology and pharmaceutical technology (IJPPT), 2012, 1(1): 53-57.

2. Kulishov S.K., Iakovenko O.M., Shvedenko A.G., Shaposhnyk O.A., Kudria I.P., Bublyk O.O. Aging as result of racemic oxymoron, fractal and anti-fractal, Moebius strip like processes. Poltava, ResearchGate, 2018, 75 p.

3.Nicki R.Colledge, Brian R. Walker, Stuart H. Ralston Davidson's Principles & Practice of Medicine. 21st Edition, Churchill Livingstone Elsevier, London, 2010, 17-38.

4. Shaver C. An Exploration of the Cantor Set. Rockhurst University .09, James and Elizabeth Monahan Summer Research Fellowship, Summer 2008, MT4960: Mathematics Seminar, Spring, 2009, 19 p.

5.Bobrov V.A., Kulishov S.K. The adaptive ischemic and reperfusion syndromes in the patients with ischemic heart disease: mechanisms, diagnosis, substantiation of therapy. Poltava: Dyvosvit, 2004, 240 p.

6.Kulishov S.K, Shtompel P.S. Mathematical modeling, programming algorithms for diagnosis of ischemic adaptation and reperfusion syndromes at patients with coronary heart disease. Materials of All-Ukrainian Congress of Ist "Medical informatics and biological informatics and cybernetics" with international participation, Proceedings, 23-26 June 2010, Kyiv, 2010, 230.

7.Kulishov S.K, Shtompel P.S. Selection principles of fractal sets for differential analysis of the systemic hemodynamic response to the test with compression-decompression of extremities at the patients with coronary heart disease. Materials of All-Ukrainian Congress of Ist "Medical informatics and biological informatics and cybernetics" with international participation, Proceedings, 23-26 June 2010, Kyiv, 2010, 231.

8.Kulishov S.K., Iakovenko O.M., Tretiak N.G. Clinical thinking training as a derivative of system and antisystem comparison, precondition to increase creativity of medical students, physicians", Proceedings of the ICL conference, (Hasselt, Belgium), 15.09.- 17.09.2010, the Kassel University Press, 2010, 337-343.

9.Kulishov S., Iakovenko O.M. Solving clinical problems using system and anti-system comparison, graphic modeling. Innovative Medicine and Biology, Canadian International Monthly Reviewed Journal (CIJIMB), ISSN 1925-2188; 2011, 3: 30-42.

10.Kulishov S., Vakulenko K., Latoha I. Myocardial electrical instability as the derivative of inflammation consumption of antiiflammatory factors syndrome, changes in geometry depolarization of atria, ventricles in the patients with coronary heart disease. Absract book of "Rhythm 2011", Congress, 2011, 39.

11.Kulishov S., Kudria I. "Stress and inflammation as determinative factors in the patients with coronary heart disease and essential hypertension", Final programme& Abstract Book of the European

Conference, IInd edition "Heart, Vessels & Diabetes", 3-5
November, Athens, Greece, 2011, 50.

12.Kulishov S., Iakovenko O.M. Individual diagnostic value of
monitoring blood glucose and arterial pressure in the patients
with diabetes mellitus and essential hypertension: a case report.
Final programme& Abstract Book of the European Conference. IInd
edition "Heart, Vessels & Diabetes", 3-5 November, Athens,
Greece, 2011, 51.

2.2. Genetic algorithm for making pharmacotherapy decisions

Prerequisites the application of genetic algorithm for making
treatment decisions in the patients with multimorbidity [1,2]

The decisive argument using genetic algorithms is closely related
to the question of how the search space is explored [1,2,3]. If this
space is easy to analyze and its topology allows the use of
specialized search technology, the use of genetic algorithms is not
efficient in terms of cost of computing resources [1,2,3]. If the
search space can not be analyzed and structured enough, and if
there is an effective method of genetic mapping of this space, the
genetic algorithm is surprisingly impressive search method in large
and complex areas [1,2,3].

Matthew Wall [1,2,4] was initiated of genetic algorithm library
(GALib). It may help us in transformation of the optimal
intermediate decisions in the final creative diagnostic and
treatment decisions [1,2].

Genetic algorithm is used for solving different problems that do
not have the solutions for the exhaustive search for polynomial
time [1,2]. Therefore, it is evolutionary calculations, i.e. genetic
algorithm preferably used in making diagnostic and therapeutic
decisions [1,2,5,6].

The modern world, highly developed industrial countries, pay attention to the problem of multimorbidity [1,2]. The main reason for this attention is the aging of populations, an increasing of the life expectancy, the number of old people and long-livers in the age structure of the population [1,2,7].

Multimorbidity is an integrated systems state to perturbation and feedback of the person's genomic, proteomic, metabolomic, neuroendocrine, immune and bioenergetics networks [1,2,8]. An integrated understanding of multimorbidity invites health professionals to consider the multiple consequences of any biomedical intervention and underscores the potential beneficial effects of implementing stress-reducing biobehavioural interventions for patients and communities alike [1,2,8].

Comorbidity and multimorbidity represent one of the greatest challenges to academic medicine [1,2,9]. Many disorders are often comorbid expressed in diverse combinations [1,2,9]. In clinical practice comorbidity and multimorbidity are underrecognized, underdiagnosed, underestimated and undertreated [1,2,9]. Comorbidities and multimorbidities are indifferent to medical specializations, so the integrative and complementary medicine is an imperative in the both education and practice [1,2,9].

Shifting the paradigm from vertical/mono-morbid interventions to comorbidity and multimorbidity approaches enhances effectiveness and efficiency of human resources utilization [1,2,9]. Comorbidity and multimorbidity studies have been expected to be an impetus to research on the validity of current diagnostic systems as well as on establishing more effective and efficient treatment including individualized and personalized pharmacotherapy [1,2,9].

Purpose of our investigation was to propose and verify the algorithm for making pharmacotherapy decision in the patients with multimorbidity [1,2].

The methodology of applying genetic algorithm for making treatment decisions in the patients with multimorbidity [1,2]

There are standards for the treatment of concrete diseases, but we have problems [1,2] with multimorbidity [10,11,12,13,14,15]. Treatment program for the patients with multimorbidity must be without polypharmacy, without iatrogenic origin pathology [1,2,10,14].

Based on these data, we considered the possible application of genetic algorithm formulation of patient treatment programs with multimorbidity based on existing standards for monomorbid cases [1,2,14]. Thus, it is necessary to make a population, each person which represents a variant of treating a patient with certain pathology [1,2]. Chromosome of this variant is composed from five genes, where each gene is certain group of drugs [1,2]. Considered to that the application of more than 5 drugs dramatically increases the risk of iatrogenic, medical complications, disease, based on these provisions, and it was proposed to limit the genes on chromosome by 5 [1,2,14]. The goal of treatment is to achieve a compiling of individual treatment regimens multimorbid states that were selected medications without contraindications to their use for each component of the multimorbidity [1,2]. Ideally, after the chosen child-chromosome genes with 5 groups of drugs need to think about the possible reduction of medication as a result of mutations up to monotherapy [1,2].

The sequence of solutions of this problem comes down to the selection of drugs for the di-morbid conditions as the descendants of mono-morbidity [1,2]. At the next stage of selection continues the most successful combinations of drugs for multimorbid states as descendants di-morbid and monomorbid states [1,2]. When breeding pairs must take into account the mutual potentiating pathogenic and / or sanogenetic effects [1,2,14]. Selection of following pairs is based on the rating of the treatment schemes, which focuses on the synergistic effects on multimorbidity processes, multi syndrome effect on each drug "gene" [1,2,14].

After the selection of the optimal therapeutic solutions of multimorbidity concrete state can be carried out to check the quality of selection at the level of the constituent syndromes [1,2].

Implementation of genetic algorithm for making diagnosis and treatment decisions

The formal-logical solutions aim of differentiation treatment multimorbid states in accordance with existing standards for optimizable and competing criteria are [1,2]:

• minimizing errors of group drugs inclusion with absolute and may be relative contraindicated for use;

• The lowest total of selected drugs with maximum therapeutic effect.

The essence of good prescribing is to pick the most appropriate drug for the disease in question, taking pathophysiology in account [1,2]. Drugs act on a wide variety of targets: receptors, transport processes, enzymes, by others miscellaneous effects [1,2]. Following administration, disposition of drugs in the body is determined by drug absorption, distribution, metabolism and excretion [1,2]. Taken together, these processes define pharmacokinetics of drug. Drug therapy monitoring, also known as Therapeutic Drug Monitoring, is a means of monitoring drug levels in the blood [1,2].

Conclusion: Thus, the criteria for the selection and evaluation are the number of syndromes and diseases in which will be to determine the best group of drugs without absolute contraindications and minimal level with relative contraindication [1,2]. More points of optimality criterions are the termination of breeding, the possibility to improve the quality of care and life [1, 2].

Genetic algorithm for making pharmacotherapy decision in the patients with multimorbidity showed effectiveness of drugs choosing [1,2].

References

1. Bobyryov V. M., Kulishov S.K., Vakhnenko A. V., Vlasova O.V. Genetic algorithm for making pharmacotherapy decision in the patients with multimorbidity. Wiad Lek, 2017; 71, 6 cz. I: 1142-1145

2. Kulishov S.K., Iakovenko O.M., Shvedenko A.G., Shaposhnyk O.A., Kudria I.P., Bublyk O.O. Aging as result of racemic oxymoron, fractal and anti-fractal, Moebius strip like processes. - Poltava, ResearchGate, 2018, 75 p.

3.De Jong K.A., Spears W. Introduction to the second special issue on genetic algorithms. Machine Learning, 1991; 5(4): 351-353.

4.Wall M. GAlib: A C++ Library of Genetic Algorithm Components, 1996.

5.Kulishov S.K. Genetic algorithm by fractal and anti-fractal exploratory analysis. Clifford Analysis, Clifford Algebras and Their Applications, 2014; 3(3): 239-248.

6.Kulishov S.K., Iakovenko O.M.: The combination of on-line and off-line learning of genetic algorithm application in diagnostic and therapeutic decision making in internal medicine clinic. Proceedings of the ninth international conference "New Information Technologies in Education for All", 2014, 25-26 November, Ukraine, Kyiv, 2014, 287-291.

7. Bezrukov V.V., Yena L.M. Multimorbidity as a problem of aging (review of literature); Problems of Aging and Longevity 2014; 23(3): 262-274.

8. Sturmberg J.P., Bennett J.M., Martin C.M., Picard M. 'Multimorbidity' as the manifestation of network disturbances. Journal of Evaluation in Clinical Practice 2016; DOI: 10.1111/jep.12587.

9. Jakovljević M. & Ostojić L. Comorbidity and multimorbidity in medicine today: challenges and opportunities for brining separated branches of medicine closer to each other. Medicina Academica Mostariensia, 2013; 01(01): 18-28.

10.Kulishov S.K., Iakovenko O.M. A combination of ischemic heart disease, diabetes mellitus type 2, and pancreatobiliary pathology: age aspects, trigger factors, and treatment of multimorbidity (review of literature and own data). Problems of Aging and Longevity, 2006; 15(3): 263-281.

11.Kulishov S. K., Vorobjov Ye. A., Novak O. V., Tretyak N. G., Savchenko , Kiryan Ye. A. Diagnostics of individual mechanisms of pathogenesis of cardiovascular and digestive pathology combined with diabetes mellitus type 2 in patients of various age. Problems of Aging and Longevity, 2007; 16(1): 41-48.

12.Kulishov S.K., Iakovenko O.M. Solving clinical problems using system and anti-system comparison, graphic modeling. Innovative medicine and biology, 2011; No 3: 30-42.

13.Kulishov S.K., Iakovenko O.M. Individual diagnostic value of monitoring blood glucose and arterial pressure in the patients with diabetes mellitus and essential hypertension: a case report. Final programme & Abstract Book of the European Conference, 2nd edition "Heart, Vessels & Diabetes", 2011 3-5 November, Athens, Greece, 2011, 51.

14. Kulishov S.K., Iakovenko O.M. Modeling Monitoring Of Age Dependent Diseases as A reflection Of Aging Genes Expressing. International Journal of Modeling and Optimization 2013; 3(1): 25-29.

15.Kulishov S., Iakovenko O., Prikhodko N., Tretiak N., Sulaiman M. Multimorbidity in the patients with diabetes mellitus and arterial hypertension as basis for dificulties in diagnostics and treatment. Programme& Abstracts of The 4th World Congress on Controversies to Consensus in Diabetes, Obesity and Hypertension; 2012, 8-11 November, Barcelona, Spain, 2011, P. 19A

Chapter 3. Perspectives of applied mathematics implementations for oxymoron like pathology diagnosis and treatment making decisions, and training

3.1. Perspectives of applied mathematics implementations for diagnosis and treatment of oxymoron like pathology

We used mathematical transformations of biomedical data as basis for exploratory analysis, creative solutions as derivatives of selective multiple testing. It's known, that subgroup analyses involve splitting all the participant data into subgroups, often so as to make comparisons between them [1,2]. Subgroup analyses may be done for subsets of participants, or for subsets of studies [1,2]. Subgroup analyses may be done as a means of investigating heterogeneous results, or to answer specific questions about particular patient groups, types of intervention or types of study [1,2]. It's known the case-based approach for characterizing and analyzing subgroup patterns as techniques for retrieving characteristic factors and cases, and merge these into prototypical cases for presentation to the user [1,2]. This method give possibilities present an alternative view on the subgroup pattern, and enable a convenient retrieval of interesting (meta-) information associated with the subgroup objects [1,2].

We proposed and tested an algorithm of using fractal and antifractal oxymorons, Moebius strip like transformations of biomedical data for exploratory subgroup analysis [2].

The algorithm is reduced to [2]:

•   initialization of study objects with fractal and antifractal data, Moebius strip like structure;

•   formation of categorical variabilities that consist from informative numeric variabilities as sum of progradient and antigradient data, including similar to "superior and inferior surfaces of strip", by iteration process as for receiving fractal and antifractal sets;

• statistical analysis of categorical variabilities and dependent numeric variabilities, using parametric and nonparametric methods;

• formulation of the conclusion.

Statistical analysis of categorical variabilities and dependent numeric variabilities as derivatives of selective multiple testing [3] included:

A. Initial selection of multiple testing methods

A1. Selection of independent and dependent variability; Calculating the of mean, standard error of mean, standard deviation, 95% confidence interval for mean, median, minimum, maximum, range, quartiles; Determination of the variabilities distribution - parametric or nonparametric by single-factor the Kolmogorov-Smirnov test; Shapiro-Wilk W test and graphical methods: frequency distribution histograms stem & leaf plots; scatter plots; box & whisker plots; normal probability plots: PP and QQ plots; graphs with error bars (Graphs: Error Bar).

A2. ANOVA (Analysis of Variance) test is used for parametric variabilities distribution. If deviations are homogeneous by Levene test would used the method of multiple comparison groups by Tukey HSD, Scheffe, Bonferroni, and in the cases without homogeneity we must use the criteria Tamhane's T2, Games-Howell;

Kruskal-Wallis test, nonparametric equivalent of the ANOVA, is used for nonparametric variabilities distribution;

A3. The selection of variabilities, as criteria for making decisions, with P = .05 or less, and / or minimal false discovery rate, q-value [4]. Determination of the sensitivity and specificity of these variabilities.

B. Secondary screening the variabilities for multiple test methods.

B1. These numerical dependent variabilities with P = .05 or less, and / or minimal false discovery rate, with high sensitivity and specificity by diagnostic capabilities must use for formation of new variabilities as descendants of 2, 3, 4 .. n numerical dependent variabilities as the derivatives of various mathematical transformations as Cantor, Sierpinski, von Koch sets, etc., anti-fractal sets; Moebius strip like aggregates, oxymoron combinations [2] and others mathematical transformations derivatives.

C. Check the newly formed variabilities similar to step A to estimate the effectiveness of such changes.

D. Comparison of multiple testing of more informative primary and secondary variabilities by accuracy, sensitivity and specificity of diagnostic possibilities.

E. If it's necessary, the search of new selection principles of variabilities for multiple testing must be continued.

Our algorithms may help to uncover underlying "re-entry" mechanisms of pathology, principles of prophylaxis and treatment oxymoron like pathology.

References

1. Atzmueller M., Puppe F. Case-based characterization and analysis of subgroup patterns. Proc. LWA, 2006, KDML Special

Track, Hildesheimer Informatik Berichte, University of Hildesheim, 2006.

2. Kulishov S.K., Iakovenko O.M.   Fractal and antifractal oxymorons, Moebius strip like transformations of biomedical data as basis for exploratory subgroup analysis. Book of abstract of International Conference on Trends and Perspective in Linear Statistical Inference; LinStat, 2014, Linkoping, Sweden, August 24-28, 2014; 58.

3. Kulishov S.K. Creative solutions as derivatives of selective multiple testing. Booklet.- CIRM CONFERENCE Mathematical Methods of Modern Statistics, France, Luminy, 10th to 14th July 2017, 21-22.

4. Gyorffy B, Gyorffy A, Tulassay Z. The problem of multiple testing and its solutions for genom-wide studies. Orv Hetil, 2005; 146 (12): 559-563.

3.2. Perspectives of GeoGebra system using for training to oxymoron like pathology diagnosis and treatment

Some of mathematical systems as GeoGebra, Tecplot, Maple, Mathematica, Matlab and others [1] may be basis for high quality of medical training.

Creative thinking of future specialists may be the result of solving heuristics, research and application tasks by Dynamic Mathematics GeoGebra [1].

The purpose of our research is to optimize the application of computer mathematical technologies to achieve professionalism;

development initiative, creative thinking; ability to apply theoretical knowledge in practice [1].

GeoGebra is the possibility of building symmetrical geometric figures relative to the coordinate axes, constructing symmetrical rotations around a point, parallel transfer of objects, use homothetic transformation, building dynamic graphics and animation creation [1,2].

The use of 3D-graphics system GeoGebra facilitates the creation and transformation of the basic model of spatial objects, performance sections of polyhedra planes, calculating the volume and surface area of polyhedrons and rotation bodies, measuring distances and angles, shapes construction of scans [1,2].

One of the criteria for student learning is to develop research competence, which includes a set of knowledge and skills required for the research, which appears in the theoretical literacy, possession of methods of psychological and educational research, the ability to statistically work out the empirical data, draw conclusions and present research results [1,2].

During the research student must use a number of stages [1]:

- observation of facts, events, staging events and issues;

- the ability to realize the problem and formulate its own; express intuitive assumptions, predictions, formulating hypotheses;

- selection of methods of testing hypotheses;

- organize special observations and experiments;

- the ability chosen methods of selection and validation, and interpretation of relevant hypotheses;

- practical conclusions and final adoption of a working hypothesis;

- control test of individual stages of studies.

GeoGebra Dynamic mathematics can promote the ability to independently acquire knowledge to diagnose and treat of oxymoron like pathology [1].

References

1. Kulishov S.K., Iakovenko O.M. GEOGEBRA system using for creative adoption of diagnostic, therapeutic decisions in internal medicine, cardiology. Presentation,· December 2016, At: Kyiv, Ukraine, Conference: Eleventh International Conference "New Information Technologies in Education for All» (ITEA-2016), 16 December 2016, e-edition: ReseachGate, 2017, DOI: 10.13140/RG.2.2.11918.15686

2.Grybyuk O.O. Mathematical modeling as a means and method of problem solving in teaching subjects of branches of mathematics, biology and chemistry. Proceedings of the First International conference on Eurasian scientific development. «East West» Association for Advanced Studies and Higher Education GmbH. Vienna, 2014, 46-53.

Author:

Kulishov Sergii Kostyantynovych

professor, Ph.D., D. Sci.

Higher State Educational Institution of Ukraine "Ukrainian Medical Stomatological Academy"

Office address: department of internal medicine No 1, HSEIU "Ukrainian Medical Stomatological Academy", street Shevchenko, 23, Poltava, Ukraine, 36011;

Email: kulishov@meta.ua;

kulishov.sergii8@gmail.com

www.ingramcontent.com/pod-product-compliance
Lightning Source LLC
Chambersburg PA
CBHW051324220526
45468CB00004B/1489

* 9 7 8 1 7 2 4 6 7 7 4 1 9 *